THE ABSENCE OF THE DEAD IS THEIR WAY OF APPEARING

MARY WINFREY TRAUTMANN

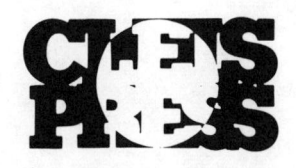

CHEMS PRESS

Copyright 1984 by Mary Winfrey Trautmann

All rights reserved. Except for brief passages quoted in newspaper, magazine, radio or television review, no part of this book may be reproduced in any form or by any means, electronic or mechanical, including photocopying or recording, or by any information storage or retrieval system, without permission in writing from the Publisher.

Published in the United States by Cleis Press, PO Box 8933, Pittsburgh, PA 15221 and PO Box 14684, San Francisco, CA 94114.

First Edition. First Printing.

Cover design: Deborah del Castillo
Cover production: Denise Dale
Typesetting: Community Press, San Francisco
ISBN: 0-939416-04-2
LC: 83-62665

Printed in the United States.

The title of this book is a paraphrase inspired by a passage in the work of Simone Weil.

This book is available on tape from the Womyn's Braille Press, PO Box 8475, Minneapolis, MN 55408.

To Carol's sisters

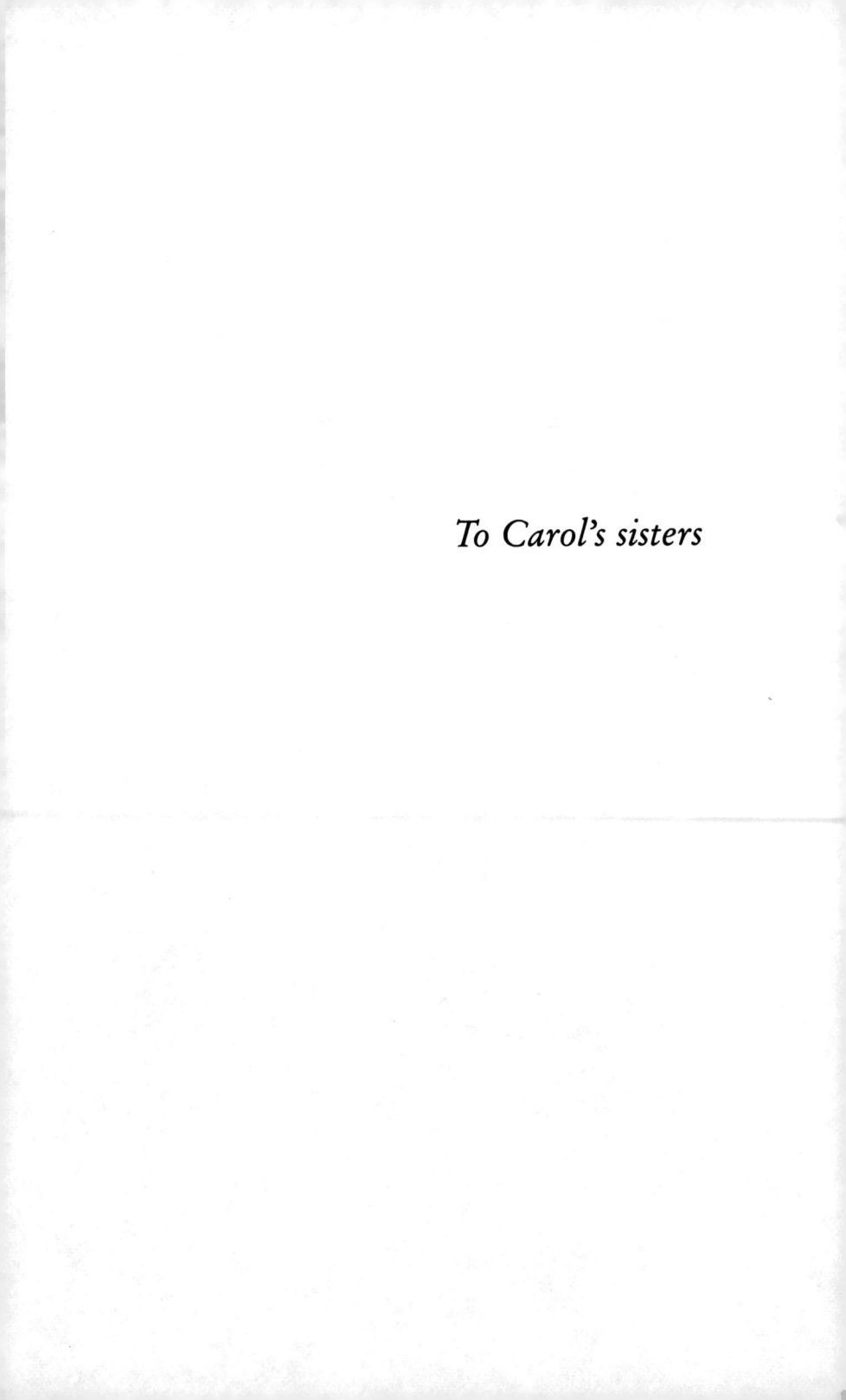

"the absence of the dead...is their way of appearing"
—Simone Weil

    if I probe with a darning needle
    and unseam the mountains
    examine what lies beneath
    the pines and caves

    if I travel darkness
    as gratefully as daylight
    talk to the wind
    drink from the flux of glaciers

    read by the radiance from planets
    sing in the deaf ravines
    dance with stones
    I have good reason:

    where you are not
    you are
    and in such roundabout measures
    I take the direct path to you

Chapter 1

It is a spring like no other, erratic and wild, blustering with tumult. In May wind and rain swirl; a heavy branch breaks from the top of the silk oak tree and shatters across the front yard. "That came close, didn't it?" I say to my husband as we pick up fragments of bark and splintered wood. I think back to January, the very start of 1973, the days sheeted with rain, the long unusually wet winter for California, the sudden lurch into spring.

Carol has been watching us from the house. She comes outside to help. Her bedroom lies under the silk oak's restless branches and she is thoroughly alarmed. "Keep calm, Carol," Paul advises. "One tree limb doesn't make a cyclone."

The rain persists and then a great many flowers and fruit trees bloom all at once—the two-toned ornamental peach, purple jacaranda, the neighbor's white magnolia, a host of red and orange hibiscus and oleander, until the bright rioting colors seem to be running a race. High flowering and gusts of wind, of course, bring the fine drifting pollen which causes Carol to sneeze and cough. She has been coughing a long time, I reflect uneasily, taking solace in the fact that a local doctor has prescribed an asthma drug for her, a fluid which she drinks daily. Still, the cough continues.

Carol does not want to see another doctor. She knows she is allergic to a large number of epidermals; this is nothing to become excited about. She is planning a beach trip with her club friends, accumulating stewpans and long-stemmed spoons. It is her responsibility, she explains with mild self-satisfaction, to bring down enough cooked food for everyone on the first night and sufficient supplies to last through the succeeding two days and nights.

Carol, who is completing her junior year at Whittier High School, has learned to manage a lathe and can manipulate tools as readily as a needle and thread; but her most recent enthusiasm is cooking. Courses like Advanced Foods and Coed Cooking are stimulating her to search expansively through newspapers and old recipe books. "You see, mom, I'm really serious about school now," she tells me pinning another of her dough-spotted underlined recipes to the bulletin board. "Aren't you glad?"

On the first night of Easter vacation she carries a simmering casserole for twenty girls to the beach, positioning the dish beside her in the car and watching over it with a wary eye. When she returns in a few days I am truly alarmed. She has lost weight, is still coughing. Her light skin has paled to alabaster, the brown eyes are puzzled, secretive. I decide to take her to an allergist at once.

Years ago when she was barely seven, Carol underwent a battery of tests, some 250 separate injections, and was found to be allergic to almost everything in the world except newsprint and kleenex and ink. For a couple of years she submitted to regular shots of antigens, then quite precipitously, quit them. She could handle the matter herself, she told me firmly, adding, "I'm sure I'm going to out-grow this junk." And her prediction seemed true enough. Now, though, this particular windy spring, I tell myself it is absolutely necessary to re-evaluate the allergy picture. She may be compelled to renew the shots whether she likes the idea or not. Adolescence, I remind myself, quoting from the universal lexicon that all mothers seem to read, adolescence is a time of serious stress.

Just before the trip to the allergist Paul asks me whether Carol is "on anything" as he obliquely puts it. She stood outside his shop door talking one afternoon, turned and stumbled. I tell him not to worry; the doctor will have an explanation. On the way to the allergist's office Carol, who insists upon driving, swerves unexpectedly, narrowly misses a collision with another car. While we wait to hear the results of her laboratory tests, Carol becomes dizzy and vomits into a basin. I suspect pneumonia, anemia, bronchitis. But no one will tell me anything; no one feels equal to telling me or my daughter the truth. I cannot discover just what it is the laboratory tests have revealed. Rather, I am met by evasions and apologies: "This isn't my field.... Why don't you see so-and-so?"

Our family physician, clearly shocked by some news bulletin we do not possess, insists that Carol enter the hospital immediately. Here in the impersonal setting of the Intercommunity Hospital we find a man who does speak out the truth—coldly and harshly, as if he takes a perverse gratification in announcing disaster. He is a specialist, a hematologist, who has seen many slides like Carol's and knows what they mean. And by now he not only has blood tests to refer to, but the irrefutable results of a bone marrow test as well.

To my husband and me he says, "No good white cells left, to speak of. Very little chance...Maybe she will be admitted to the City of Hope, I'll try.... If they are studying her particular kind of leukemia, they may accept her as a patient." It is Sunday when he utters these words. May 13. Mothers' Day.

In our mutual shock Paul and I cannot protest his harshness which derives, I sense, from too many years of dealing with this special form of white death; years of facing too many parents who want reassurance and hope when there is none to give. A purveyor of bad news and sorrow, he has almost no human warmth left. I, of course, hate him and then in time forgive him.

Our daughter is accepted by the national medical and research center at Duarte, California, which is called the City of Hope. Carol, her family and her numerous friends, begin to acquaint themselves with Wing Five, the hematology section of this large complex. It is Paul who abruptly suggests that I write out the story of Carol, saying on the evening of the third day after we learn she has somehow contracted acute myeloblastic leukemia—our second child and only sixteen years old—"Well, you consider yourself something of an author, you've published, why don't you write about all this? Who knows, it might be quite a story...."

He says these words in a moment of enthusiasm, after we have listened to all the happy endings well-intentioned people relate to suddenly stricken parents. It is after Mrs. Alfredo visits Carol's room, number 531 at the City of Hope, and, standing carefully out of our daughter's hearing range, announces: "Take courage...Believe me, I know a young woman with leukemia, she has had it now for ten years and, you know what, she is married and has children yet! There are wonderful, wonderful kinds of treatment these days. Your daughter is in the best of hands!"

How we both love Mrs. Alfredo! How eagerly we help her search the corridors for her son's room! He, too, has leukemia, chronic, she says briefly, adding in semi-dark tones that he has over-strained himself, is too tired, low-spirited, in danger of giving up. As it turns out, we never do identify Mrs. Alfredo's son. We leave her in a room occupied by several young men, all with pallid faces, wearing a look of boredom and hopelessness, resigned patience, an expression we feel confidently will never mar the brightness of our daughter's face.

There is an initial period of adjustment; it is like having to move to a foreign country, re-locating. Everyone commends the attractiveness of the hospital grounds, the immaculate well-appointed rooms; praises the doctors, the technology we are surrounded by. Carol does not yet know how ill she is. We all shield her.

Chemotherapy has started. Paul and I sign a paper authorizing the use of daunomycin, which is a new anti-leukemic drug, deep red in color like burgundy wine and producing strong nausea. Cytosine is combined with this powerful drug. At some point a third medication, thioguanine, is added, taken orally in tablet form.

Dr. Graham is Carol's doctor. She has lived in Jamaica and studied at McGill University in Canada, but is actually Lebanese, I think. She tells me my daughter has a fifty percent chance of ever gaining remission. I am numb, merely stare at her. Dr. Graham says, as if astonished, "But surely you know WHAT THIS IS don't you?"

As it happens, I do not know, though I am gradually learning that Carol's situation is different from that of the chronic leukemic patient: more complex, I sense, more immediately hazardous. My store of medical knowledge is scant, my attitude unscientific. The few articles and newspaper paragraphs I have read are certainly inadequate; yet I do not intend to become an authority on Carol's leukemia. Intuitively, I desire to keep all bitter informants at bay, to study no discouraging life expectancy charts or bleak percentages. My attitude is in defiance of medicine and statistics, perhaps, reason. My one clear inner resolve is to stay close to Carol, to see this thing through with her no matter what consequences follow.

Dr. Graham finds Paul objective and lucid. Listening to them talk, I learn several new facts almost against my will: *One,* Carol, medically speaking, occupies a nebulous borderline between the child and the adult. The medical team at first considered giving her the treatment that is normally reserved for children, then abandoned the idea. *Two,* the illness behaves erratically, can result in a rapid proliferation of white cells or, as now, the reverse, an extremely low count. *Three,* Carol, once in remission, has a short life expectancy, two years at the most. *Four,* among patients who have her type of acute leukemia, a small *one percent* recovers completely. This is called natural remission or a miracle. Paul and I clutch this tantalizing statistic. We are determined that Carol will fall within the scope of the one percent, we embrace the miracle. Dr. Graham is silent.

Paul cancels his scheduled trip to Italy and England. He manages an electronics company in the City of Industry and the pressures on him are steadily accelerating. Business meetings and trips consume more and more of his time and I, in a moment of frustration, accuse him of "hiding out in his precious factory," a remark that leads to recriminations and to my tears. He has his own way of handling the tensions that are tearing at us both. But I realize he can escape into a world of business and practical affairs, a thing I cannot do. "Men are not bound, as women are, to the world of blood and birth and cycles. To be a woman is like living your life swimming under water..." I cannot remember who said these words originally, what writer I am unconsciously quoting. I feel myself inexorably concentrating on my daughter; the intensity of this focusing causes me physical pain. My life slows down to stay in step with hers. At moments I am subject to sudden uncontrollable impulses, reach out to stroke her arm or smooth her hair. But even these gestures are contained within a gradually slowing rhythm.

Yes, I am living under water, swimming through the heavy opaque fluid that presses in on every side.

Chapter 2

The days waver by. When Paul visits the City of Hope on his lunch hour or at night, just before treatment, accompanied by Julie, Carol's fourteen-year-old sister, he acts cheerful, can often behave as if the leukemia were basically a chimera, a bad nightmare which has agreed to vanish at some undisclosed moment. He jokes, teases Julie, says to Carol: "Hey, Car-olee-o, what's the latest hot scoop on the news, what's Nixon been up to?" Toying with the mechanisms in the room, he lightly touches the controls that raise and lower the bed and states, "I'll bet you don't even know who designed these contraptions," and we hear again the story of Howard Hughes and the evolution of the modern hospital bed. Carol begins to glow, a camaraderie is established. Then a nurse enters to start an I.V. and she grabs my fingers.

By now we realize that her veins are small and difficult to locate. We are compelled to concentrate on a matter none of us has ever considered before—the size and availability of veins. "But I think of them all the time, I honestly do," a young nurse confides to me. She is constantly studying the blood vessels in other people's forearms, she says, glancing at my wrists. My eyes follow hers; the pulsating cords I see travelling down my arms would obviously be easy to pierce. Compared to mine Carol's veins are like slim blue threads.

The night Carol's first I.V. is administered we meet a number of nurses and aides who come in and out of the room to assist, women that we think of as hospital friends: the equable Mrs. Golley, Mrs. Knoke, always referred to as "Birdie," Jill March, Cathy Robinson, the soft-spoken Mrs. De Leera. The butterfly needles the nurses use are aptly named; they are narrow-bodied, winged, unpredictable. The first injections grope, withdraw, leave a splotch beneath the skin on Carol's right wrist. Finally one of the winged needles alights properly. The fluids descend from their inverted bottles, the I.V. proceeds. And Carol, left with the purple blotch which fades but does not go away, puts on long sleeves, tries to camouflage the embarrassment at her wrist however she can. Someone refers to the bruising as a hematoma, saying the vein has collapsed here and cannot be used again, but later on I am told this is inaccurate—a true hematoma is a tumor.

It is only the start, the first series of treatments, and Carol cannot resist playing practical jokes now and again. One night after Paul arrives and the I.V. stand is wheeled in, she fakes a cry of pain, holds the back of her hand to her mouth in an attitude of despair, creates a flurry, so that the nurses gather around the bed like a host of fidgety bees. Nothing whatsoever has happened. "You just don't know this girl yet, nurse!" Paul exclaims, while Carol continues to improvise, extending her little drama until she explodes with mirth.

The next day I see her stun a group of awe-struck friends by placing her hands on her throat in a pose worthy of Bette Davis and declaiming huskily, "I've only got two more weeks." She settles back to watch everyone's reactions, wide-eyed, a small observant sphinx. It is absurd, pure teen-age soap opera—excruciating, lethal.

Before the series concludes the hematology team made up of Dr. Graham and three male colleagues interrogates Carol during a "grand round" of Wing Five. Carol studies the specialists carefully while they are analyzing her; I feel certain that after they leave she intends to entertain Paul and me with a comic sketch of her four inquisitors. "Yes," she admits under their scrutiny and questions, "yes, I have noticed the lesions on my back and hips, too. Loss of weight, yes." Paul and I listen, discover more details, learn of new symptoms. She has been aware of the red dots on her skin for several weeks, conscious, also, of a too-rapid heart-beat." And have you had any problems with vision, Carol?" one of the men asks. Again the answer is "yes."

These are intimations and warnings which Carol has been disregarding. At sixteen she cannot take such cryptic signals seriously. She surrounds herself with joy and friendliness, walks in an aura of sunlight. It is easy to laugh; a fresh joke, a hoary pun, a bird tangling thread in its beak, her dog worrying a rag, the pomposity of a hospital, can cause a rivulet of laughter to escape from her, a sound, one of the nurses whispers to me, that the whole staff delights in hearing. They do not mind her practical jokes, they all love Carol.

It is less easy to laugh when the nausea comes at night following treatment, with a remorselessness she will never discuss. In the morning we see the untouched food, the listlessness, the dawdling over breakfast for hours before she at last requests a milk-shake or limeade from the small kitchen around the corner. She saves rolls and hard-boiled eggs for Julie and me. She smiles when she hears my anecdote about her latest breakfast egg, the one that turned out to be soft-boiled, how it rolled and squashed all day inside my purse. "The yolk was on you, wasn't it, mother?" she says.

Carol shrugs at the festive-looking trays that are brought over regularly from the main cafeteria. "Bring me a big dill pickle from the German delicatessen, will you please, mother?" she pleads or else asks, "Have the birds left any apricots on the tree at the top of the hill?" I carry paper bags filled with oranges and apricots and store them in the kitchen cubicle on Wing Five. I place enormous green pickles immersed in pickle juice and secured by plastic envelopes beside Carol's tray.

The main cafeteria, set among trees and pink floral borders, can be reached in a few minutes after leaving the Wing. Tall shrubs only partially veil the standing walls which are an integral part of the landscaping; the walls are monuments covered with plaques which are engraved with the names of donors. Memorials lurk everywhere at the City of Hope, people's names are written on many surfaces in gardens and lounges and waiting rooms. I idly take to reading the plaques, assigning personalities and histories to the individual names, reconstructing cities and towns in my imagination. The cafeteria with its memorabilia establishes itself as one of the stations I frequent during my daily pilgrimages.

Is Carol responding to treatment? Is her bone marrow making any white cells? Is she better, IS SHE? Over and over again when I ask these questions I am told, always politely, that my daughter "continues to hold her own," a statement that frustrates analysis. It simply means that she is still alive.

Admittedly there is not enough for me to do here, yet I cannot leave the panorama of the hospital for long; I am pulled into its colorful smooth-flowing rhythms as snugly as a leaf riding into an eddy. A furious suspense grips me. I have no more strength than the leaf, I stand outside the hospital's dynamics and yet at their heart, watching, feeling time spiral in upon itself as it assumes an unknown unforeseeable contour. Nothing in my life has prepared me for this intolerable suspense, no event, conditioning or previous crisis, not childbirth not the death of either of my parents.

I invent things to do, purchase a paperback book entitled *Testimony for Man* and begin reading the history of the City of Hope. I spend an hour surveying abalone jewelry and embroidered cotton blouses in the gift shop, move across the hall to the racks of stationery and candy. It is simple enough to select brightly colored jelly beans for Carol, but what do I want, chocolate-covered peanuts or toasted coconut bars? The choice becomes fateful, overwhelming me. I cannot make up my mind. My brain seems composed of alien dry cogs that barely turn and so I decide nothing, simply buy more jelly beans.

I conceal the bewilderment which encompasses me in

ever-increasing ripples by being as functionally useful as possible. I change the water in the flower containers in Carol's room, tug the portable telephone about and take down messages. I am present, on the spot, at the moment an I.V. is begun and Carol wants to clutch me. The books I read, the letters I write, even the diary entries, are a façade concealing my actual preoccupation, the vigil that absorbs me. While Carol sleeps or watches television and the hot summer days undulate past, I observe every changing nuance of her face and body.

A student nurse, earnest and purposeful, takes me aside and says: "I don't honestly know what your relationship with your daughter is, but anyhow, perhaps when Carol sees you coming here every day she realizes you are neglecting other responsibilities and this fact," the student nurse continues firmly, "may very well add to her own feelings of depression—the withdrawal she is struggling with." She gestures toward the untouched school books which Carol has left in view. "What is here, what is she taking in school? Chemistry, history, advanced foods. Well, why not call her counselor, find a tutor, someone to renew her interest in studying? Her friends and her mother are not the—Now, when I was sixteen," she interrupts herself, getting, possibly, to the real core of the message, "at that age I could never have spoken to my mother about my feelings about myself. Perhaps she needs to be alone more, perhaps she just needs to cry."

The student nurse means to give me useful advice, some guidelines to follow, but she does not answer the questions that are obsessing me. How does anyone face death at sixteen? How is time to be gotten through? Will my daughter live?

I resolve to accept the well-meant suggestions, to leave the hospital earlier, not spend quite so many hours haunting its corners. I thank the nurse and return to Carol's bedside where I say goodbye with firmness. As I pass through the outpatient clinic, occupied now by only a few stragglers, I notice the small office of the social service department. The tall woman who emerges through the doorway looks familiar; Paul and I met her the day Carol entered the City of Hope, when we were all learning its procedures for the first time. A powerful impulse compels me to stop walking in front of a row of empty wheelchairs. Is there a course to follow and does she know the way? The tall woman hurries past, her arms filled with folders. She is unaware of my rigid pose, the vulnerability it masks. Her eyes slide over and around me. I realize she does not remember that we were ever introduced.

I turn to the right of the desk and leave.

Chapter 3

Carol is coming home. The first series of chemotherapy treatments is over. She will be allowed to take rides in automobiles and visit a few friends. If she stays in the car she can watch the lions at Lion Country Safari, Dr. Graham says.

She falls asleep almost at once on the water-bed that sits under the orange and gold flowered curtains in her bedroom. Her dog Blackie, part spaniel and part pekinese, shaggy and dark with a blaze of white on his chest and paws, keeps ferocious guard over her. He hurls himself at any person who steps too far into the room.

I walk softly, stand quietly at the entrance to the yellow bedroom, straining to see my daughter's face. I study the skin's fine transparency that reminds me of jonquil petals in spring, the faint pink flush accentuating the high cheek-bones. Are the blood transfusions responsible for this delicate blush, I wonder, and have the dark smudges beneath her eyes actually gone away?

She breathes deeply, almost luxuriously, as if savoring the air. Her long yellow hair is tossed over the pillow, the slightly parted mouth emphasizes the fullness of the lower lip. How fragile flesh and blood are, I think, and the concept of fragility in my mind transmutes her briefly into porcelain, into an exquisitely molded china figurine which might fall from the bed and break at any moment, or else return to an implacably distant pose on the lid of a music box where she revolves to a slow unearthly music outside the range of human ears. Carol smiles in her deep slumber. I am looking at flesh and blood, not porcelain, but in spite of this fact I sense a transformation occurring even as I watch, a change I cannot analyze—except to note that she seems to be growing younger. She is a child, sleeping, moving away from me, through dreams involved with mysterious transactions in which I have no part. Who is she, I ask, woman or child or figurine?

I step away from the bedroom, find my diary and begin writing. The act of writing will sustain me like the prayers I invent from time to time and whisper under my breath. The diary will clarify and refine my thoughts; it will diminish the sad faces, the suddenly dropped voices that I encounter unexpectedly when I enter a bank or grocery store, voices that enquire and want to be solicitous. Yet it is apparent that many of the people who speak to me have decided that Carol is in reality dead. I write to refute these people.

Carol is awake most of the time, not sleeping, and I, in my role of novice nurse, attempt to remind her of the precautions laid down by her doctor. She does not like even the hint of supervision. She remembers everything, she tells me shortly, and lists the medications on the bedside table—enovid, alloprinal, ampicillin, what else do I want her to take?

It is difficult to remonstrate with a combative defensive Carol. "The ampicillin, that's the antibiotic. You're supposed to have four a day," I remark. "Ampicillin will, ah, protect you from infection, won't it?"

"Yes, mom. Sure, mom. They told me that." She glares at me for a moment.

Of course she cannot see the warnings that shape themselves inside my head. *Danger. Infection.* Almost no white cells. Watch for bleeding, for sweats, chills, fever. Carol cannot hear the words, either, spoken by the hematologist at the Intercommunity Hospital on the day he identified her leukemia. "I must caution you both," he repeats brusquely to

Paul and me as we sit in the quiet hospital chapel, a dimly lighted room of dark wood and gray stone, "...parents have very special feelings about a child of this sort. A child like this," he says again. "Parents treat her differently. I want to remind you..." He breaks off, finally finishes the sentence "...not to lose perspective entirely." He stares at the wall, ignoring me.

I discover that I have no perspective to lose where Carol is concerned. She is home from the hospital at last; we allow the angry moment to ebb away, then laugh and embrace each other. We become allies and confidantes. She washes her yellow hair, happily dries it in the warm sun on the patio. "Do you think they'll find a cure for leukemia in my lifetime?" she asks. I nearly drop the platter I am carrying. "Oh, I don't think too much about the cure, really, Mom," she adds. "I just wonder how the heck I ever got it."

The two of us sit outdoors and discuss the "break-through in leukemia" that nearly everyone we know is referring to. There is little solid information, but considerable rumor, so much of it that one of Carol's teachers tells her, "Well, research is very close to finding an answer, so, Carol, if you have this thing, now is certainly the time." I mention Dr. Salk and the polio vaccine and grope for possible parallels. Leukemia must be nearing the break-through point, cancer and leukemia will soon be obsolete terms, we reassure each other, putting our heads together and talking about heredity, horse-back riding in Colorado and Vermont, the past, the future.

She is delighted to be home again. She plays with Blackie who shows off in an ecstasy of self-consciousness, jumping far higher than his usual powers permit and capturing a moth. She bakes a lemon cake, drizzling a tart sauce-like frosting on the crust, marking indentations with a fork so that the sauce will hold. She teases her sunburnt sister who returns unexpectedly from the beach. "Hey, Julie, what did you do in the kitchen last besides eat?" she challenges. Her warmth and wit dance about our heads. Her radiance enchants us. The day passes like a drop of slow golden honey.

The next morning Carol talks on the phone to her older sister Amy who is living in Milwaukee with Aunt Bea and Uncle Phil. The two sisters converse breathlessly. "But, Carol, you don't sound ill," Amy remarks.

"I'm not ill, I just have an incurable disease," she replies. It is the first time I have heard her make this statement and I cannot keep from wincing.

Dr. Graham's restrictions are forgotten as Carol inhales the heady air of freedom. She goes to school where her counselor, Mr. Leonard, states that she has been excused from finals in every class. Her work, the teachers say, is uniformly excellent. Carol is vastly pleased. Mr. Leonard does not believe she needs a tutor. He listens with approval to her plans to take oceanography, foods, public speaking and typing in the fall. Mrs. Davis, a homemaking instructor, announces that Carol will receive the outstanding student award in advanced foods. The Crisco Corporation sponsors the award, so Carol's boy friend Steve begins calling her "the Crisco Kid." She visits more classes, mingles with throngs of students in the school quad, her pleasure deepening.

While Carol is getting re-acquainted with high school, Steve's mother, Marlene Spiri, phones to ask if my daughter can be included in the Spiris' tentative plans for a trip to Mammoth and possibly a stay at the beach later on in August. "It's up to the doctor," I say. "When she's better, why yes, it's all right with me." Marlene is aware of our midwestern origins, knows that Carol has no grandmother, aunt or uncle within two thousand miles, but, she says, "...the relatives, both Jack's and mine, enjoy Carol as if she were another cousin," and then she remarks before hanging up, "I just treat her naturally these days. I hardly ever ask her how she feels any more."

Carol goes to a meeting of the Honovian Club, returning with flushed cheeks and a head filled with anecdotes, the argument still making the rounds over her leukemia and the unreliability of diagnoses, the outrageous methods her friends used to sneak passes at the hospital. "Why, we held our Monday night meeting in my room," she confesses. "There must have been thirty girls and the nurses just gave up and hid until they all went home."

Carol and I go shopping together; she buys blue jeans and a summer dress, two bow ties for her father. I ask if she is tired. "No, no!" she protests. "I don't ever want to go back to the hospital, either!" I glance at her inquiringly. "Look, I'm writing down a list of questions to ask Dr. Graham," she confides, showing me a spiral notebook. "And the first one is this: can Carol stay home all next week, please? But I've already got the answer here in large print. Dr. Graham says ABSOLUTELY NOT."

Carol goes out with Steve, stays up late to watch television with Paul. She refuses to conform to any hospital blueprint. Some of the young boys in the neighborhood that she and her sisters used to play with knock on the door. She sits with them, laughing and talking, in the front yard under the silk oak tree, Blackie beside her.

I linger in the background, try to check her temperature now and again, pursue my fleet-footed daughter like a persistent gadfly, know I will continue the pursuit all summer and longer, will accept the morose moods and the introspection gladly, hopefully, in exchange for the golden honey days, whenever they fall.

THE METRONOME

The sound is scarcely audible at first, no more than a pulse ticking away or the low thud of my own heart beat, but once I hear it during the repetitive rhythms of lap swimming, I concentrate, re-focus my senses, refine the mechanism of my inner ear until the white plastic swim cap that binds my head puts no appreciable barrier between me and the steady drumming tone. It is a metronome I am listening to, a slow-moving pendulum swinging invisibly below me underneath the waves. I identify its unseen presence, perceive the metronome clairvoyantly rather than visually, but at the same time I do not understand why I perceive it or why it should appear at all.

In my entire experience as a swimmer, whether training for amateur competitions, sprints, relays, races, or leisurely swimming distance for sheer enjoyment, I have never noticed the metronome before. Possibly it was always there, resting at the bottom of each river, lake or pool, sending its pulsations vertically through the waves as I swam, but I was deaf to its rhythms. For years I heard nothing. I do begin to hear the metronome now for the first time, during the summer I decide to take up routine distance swimming again, slipping into a pattern that is completely familiar to me, as pleasurable as glimpsing the remembered landscape of childhood.

The work-outs occur in the mornings or at noon, always at the same place, the old neighborhood pool where my three daughters learned to swim when they were very young. Abandoning the beaches and surf of the Pacific coast, I swim intensely within the confines of the small blue-tiled pool of my choice, concentrating as if I were training for a channel race. I have never been more serious about my flutter kick, the precise angle at which my arms enter the water or the momentum of their downward pull, yet engrossed as I am in physical motions and the minutiae of form, I hear the metronome in full cadence every time I reach the start of the second lap. As it ticks away I count, biting down on foam; and the counting in my head turns into words, monosyllables at first that I speak into the shallow waves, the chlorine, the motes that drift by, lazily penetrating and clouding the layers of water. The monosyllables pour out while I count and count during each successive lap, saying, for example: "*eight / eight / eight laps / wait fate,*" not particularly noticing the rhyme. My hands reach the pool's edge, my body makes the turn and I say into the small surf that my arms and legs are creating: "*nine / nine / nine / sign / send sign*" and the nonsense goes on, my legs settle into a rhythm that they find natural to them, my feet pursue their kick, kick, kick.

The laps spin past, the turns at the end of the pool repeat themselves, I mark the quarter mile, the half mile, and find that I am chanting, even shouting, into the water streaming by my eyes, floods which seem colored the hue of the pool tiles. I chant, I sing rhymes that bubble through this water and the rhymes continue to maintain a communion with the metronome at the bottom of the pool: "*forty-five, forty-five / let life live / stay alive; forty-seven, forty-seven / hear me / hear me / not be riven...*" These phrases are nothing less than an importuning from my mind and body, a supplication flung to the waves which, as the work-out ends, leaves me enervated and spent.

Sometimes, counting and chanting through the mote-filled streams, I grasp the tiled pool edge and in the moments before completing the turn and push away from the wall, I see my three small daughters swimming toward me. They are trying to capture my attention, they want to interrupt my monotonous lap swimming by clambering up on my shoulders; and just for a second our finger tips touch in the foam. Then the figures falter and slip away from me.

Sometimes there has been too much chemotherapy or too much pain. The metronome beats even more clearly then and I recognize that subtle instrument's purpose, what it has meant all along, even during the years I did not hear it. I know why it sounds so plainly now: the pendulum in motion, the drum, the gong throbbing out the inexorable beat of time that is passing for my daughter, that pulses through my own body, reverberates in the furrows of my ears, time, marking its path through the universe, departing, passing, beating, on its way to timelessness, which is a region I cannot see or hear or love.

Chapter 4

May changes to June. The war with infection accelerates, but Carol develops delaying tactics that would make any military commander proud. She learns how to mask symptoms, how to minimize and evade. "If I go to the hospital they'll keep me there," she says defiantly, putting another layer of powder over a reddened nostril.

One morning the nostril is so swollen and inflamed that I peremptorily call the City of Hope and make arrangements to take her in. We leave hurriedly, only to spend long hours sitting in the out-patient clinic. Carol picks up her file at the entrance desk, barely smiling at the woman who gives it to her. The file records every visit and hospitalization, each complete blood count and contact with a doctor; it seems thin and insubstantial compared with the files I glimpse being passed from hand to hand, the reports stapled between cardboard covers that form bulky volumes. Carol's file is like a preface to a chapter not yet written.

Carol glooms at her yellow CBC slip and frowns at the splashy bronze-toned impressionistic paintings that hang on the clinic walls flanked by gold-lettered quotations. She settles down to the pages of *Mad* magazine while I try to focus on Tolkien, who is a new author for me. Detecting a moderate curiosity in the angle of Carol's wandering gaze and tilted chin, I attempt to read a few lines of *The Hobbit* aloud to her, but am subdued by an out-pouring of patients welling into the area. They appear as if answering a summons, spread across the couches and chairs, ask for hot water, make coffee or tea at the tables set out for the purpose, preoccupy themselves with magazines or, possibly, toys, for they make up a heterogeneous group of every imaginable age and interest. I notice an infant with a shaved head who is strapped inside a stroller, a white-haired woman talking calmly through an artificial larynx. A young man falls asleep cushioned against his mother's shoulder. She stares at him with a haunted, searching look that brings a rush of emotion to my throat.

Everyone I see is different and yet, paradoxically, the same. Some inexplicable thing that has been labelled "catastrophic" causes these people to come together, to sit here composedly on the glossy couches, hour after hour, with endless patience, waiting to have blood drawn, to be weighed, and x-rayed and evaluated. They make a sociable assemblage, for the most part, are well-known to one another, spend the slowly passing time in chitchat or playing cards, now and then succumbing to drowsiness. Except for an occasional wheelchair, an artificial device carried or worn casually, they might be vacationers anticipating the arrival of a tour bus. They have learned how to wait. A monumental patience defines them all.

Carol reads two issues of *Mad* magazine and one issue of *The New Yorker* before her blood is drawn and processed. Dr. Graham wears a blue mask over her mouth and nose while she examines Carol. I wonder if the mask is necessary or if the doctor is trying to impress my high-spirited daughter with the fact of her own mortality. Perhaps it is meant as a warning: *slow down, your life is in danger, your life.*

Yes, I did the right thing in bringing her in, Dr. Graham assures me. Carol will need more medication and lots of hot compresses applied near the side of the nose. But she can probably still be treated at home. Carol, reprieved and supplied with more antibiotics, agrees. When we return to the house, eyeing each other like wary combatants under a flag of truce, Julie greets us enthusiastically. She has been swimming again;

her mahogany-red arms and legs contrast appreciably with her sister's paleness.

Carol goes quietly to her room and all at once I find myself nagging at Julie. Help! I demand of her. Give me a hand with the house, with the animals, their incessant feedings. "Why didn't you feed Mousey this morning?" I ask. "Isn't she your cat? Can't you make up a few beds, fold the laundry? Do you know how to prepare a hot compress for your sister's face?"

Julie backs away, protesting. She does not understand what a compress is. I begin a long explanation, starting with the bone marrow and its failure to produce proper white cells, the leukocytes, those invisible masses of granular tissue so necessary to the body if it is to resist infection. I switch over to the complete blood count, how it is usually broken down into three components—hemoglobin, platelets and white cells—how the typical young woman maintains a hemoglobin of 12, whereas Carol—

"Yes, yes," Julie interrupts. "I know all that. Everybody at school is talking about it. I don't hardly hear anything else. Everyone asks me how she is, how she's doing, every single day, mom."

I stop, silenced, contrite. Of course, Julie must be satiated with the subject; as a matter of fact, we all are, but no one more thoroughly than Carol herself. I make a light supper which the three of us eat quickly, as we listen to radio news bulletins and band music, John Philip Sousa, because the Fourth of July is coming. Later, sinking onto a crumpled bedspread in the back bedroom, I cry violently for a moment and then sleep.

Suddenly she is in real trouble. Her nose swells, a mushrooming pain spreads through the left side of the chest and shoulder, pains in the rib cage, difficulty with breathing, a temperature of 102 degrees. She is admitted to the City of Hope at once. But each admittance follows a specific procedure; she must sign papers in duplicate at the small central office and enter Wing Five the official way, in a wheelchair. "Sorry, Carol," the nurse says, "but it's the rule. Please just sit down."

Carol mopes but obeys, slightly mollified by the fact that her father is wheeling her chair along the green carpeted passageway. She considers the wheelchair an indignity, is accustomed to taking care of herself, walking proudly upon the sidewalk beneath the trellis with its burgeoning vines and yellow flowers, while ignoring the wheelchairs that wait bunched together within easy reach. She is used to standing in line, pale and determined, often with a hemoglobin of six or less, a white count so negligible that the nurses cannot understand where she summons up the strength for motion. Today, her father takes charge. He wheels her through the green and aqua-tinted realm of Wing Five to a spotless room where the bed sheets are folded back, the nurses, the I.V. stand, the T.V. set, are positioned and ready.

Today the City of Hope is itself in crisis, trying to cope with a power failure. Hours pass before the switch can be made from an emergency power system back to the normal one and, during the interval, no x-rays can be taken. There is no television to watch, very little hot water is available for compresses. Carol disregards the inconveniences. She seems withdrawn, self-absorbed.

The blue and green realm of Wing Five is growing more and more familiar to me. I see the hematology team of three white-coated men and one woman station themselves around Carol's bedside, witness again their polite deference and probing questions. To the medical team Carol is a study in pathology, an acute myeloblastic leukemia case, until all at once she makes them laugh and the doctors and the room are humanized, warmed with friendliness. I recognize individual faces among the aides and interns, nurses and cleaning ladies, all of whom greet me with brisk cheerfulness, as if acknowledging that the bond connecting us pulls harder now, is tightening.

Before the day is over Carol undergoes a barrage of x-rays. When she comes back from the lab, stretched out flat on a hospital gurney, she describes the over-attentive orderly who "is trying to pick up on me," as she puts it. With mingled exasperation and amusement she repeats the words he murmured in her ear, "Carol, if you ever want your back rubbed by a real man, ask for me!" We both laugh.

The new accelerating infection turns out to be pleurisy. It is useless to speculate how she contracted this or to utter reproaches. A few days pass, though, and one tense morning a real quarrel flares between us, a controversy over Senior Week, which is to begin on the following Monday. Carol wants to participate. She bombards Dr. Graham with requests. "You are a Senior then?" the doctor counters mildly, trying not to make any commitment.

"Well, no," says Carol, "not exactly, but Steve is." She is determined to savor every event during the whole week, especially graduation night. I say such a plan is impractical, she has to compromise. She will not yield a single demand. Angry words splutter to the surface where they blaze and leap until I leave the room and wander disconsolately outside on the lawns kicking at strips of bark from the peeling eucalyptus trees.

Carol leaves the Wing, too, I find out later, and also rambles through the sun-streaked gardens, but we do not meet again until evening, both of us chastened, eager for reconciliation. "Mother, I'm sorry," she says. "Carol, I'm sorry," I say at the same time.

Suddenly, as if a totally random thought has entered her mind, Carol asks, "Do you remember the boy across the hall in room 531?"

Something in her voice subdues me and I wait, not intruding my immediate recollections.

"Mother, I think he died last night. Oh, yes, I do: I think I saw it happen." She is answering the puzzlement on my face, the unspoken denials. "Birdie tried to cover it up. But everything moved so fast, she was too late. It happened right before dinner..."

"But, Carol, I was here, too," I blurt out.

"Yes. You were watching television. Your back was to the door. But I was looking and I could see him on the bed and an oxygen tent went in with a lot of people and then a stretcher and then, Mom, you know what? Birdie came in my room and asked if she could eat a peach, and shut the door. *She shut the door!*"

I continue to say nothing.

"Yesterday he talked to me," she says softly. "And he was just fine, walking around, barely even using his walker, and laughing. Do you remember how he used to eat so much?"

I nod my head, picturing the young man leaning on a modified walker, talking Spanish to the orderly; I visualize the plates heaped with tostados and rice, the flirtation tentatively begun with Carol.

"He had leukemia," she says. "And he liked me." She grows silent as if thinking about what the two of them held in common or had briefly shared—the strange unpredictable illness, the random conversations, room 531, Wing Five.

"Perhaps there were complications," I say at last. "Maybe his doctor wanted him taken to intensive care." It is the best I can do and the remark does not satisfy her. She sinks back on the pillow; I try not to dwell upon images of disaster, the chance impersonal destruction of human life, the gigantic hand that tilts a large chessboard abruptly to the vertical and sends pawns and queens alike sliding to the floor.

Moments afterward I encounter Dr. Graham at the nursing station. She informs me that the boy in room 531 did indeed die during the supper hour on the preceding night. A death on the Wing cannot be kept secret, the patients feel it, she admits with reluctance. "It's as if they all have a sixth sense and can tell when someone dies."

She waits a moment and then says, "I am surprised that Carol will not discuss this matter with me. But she won't, she doesn't say anything to the nurses either. She is keeping it to herself, suppressing the whole thing, Mrs. Trautmann."

I feel that in some obscure way I am undergoing a reprimand.

"It is better for her to ask questions," the doctor says. "She should bring her suspicions out into the open. It is better to talk about death."

I am conscious of nuance, but my senses are numbing, they are focusing elsewhere at a point outside my will and control, and I do not grasp the doctor's meanings, her expectations, do not know in what manner either Carol or I have failed her, or just how anyone discusses death with a sixteen-year-old.

"She is making platelets at last, but still practically no white cells." Dr. Graham muses. "Things are not going as well as we wish. Of course it is early yet." She pauses. "More treatment, more treatment," she repeats and then continues with a somewhat tangled statement: "We will tell Carol to do whatever she can, once she improves, and not to cut out her boy friend's graduation next week since this is so important to her—but let her do what she can, some things, some things... She is too young, of course, she does not understand what this illness means." Turning away abruptly she adds, "Teen-agers are always the worst, they do not want to accept anything."

I learn with relief that Carol can go home after she has had blood transfusions. Even under the most ideal circumstances transfusions are very slow, but tonight the red drops gathering in the plastic bags at the top of the I.V. stand wait in a kind of paralysis; they forget how to fall, once they have shaped themselves into beads. Carol rattles the plastic tubes and bags impatiently.

Hold on, blood is a thick complex substance, I tell her, and a lot can go wrong if the transfusion is made too rapidly. She answers with an angry jerk at the plastic tubing. For a moment my mind dips into fantasy, the absurdity of two teams, the red cells and the white cells, each counting off and joining their teammates on opposite sides of the I.V., the intrusion of a third group, the beige and neutral platelets, who line up between the two factions and gradually unite them until red, white and beige elongate into a pennant that flutters from the top of the metal stand.

I snap out of the fantasy. But the I.V. unit reminds me of a cross, there can be no doubt about it, and I grimly consider crucifixion, then reverse the image, the I.V stand as a cross-road, the road of life, through which travel life-perpetuating fluids: saline solution, platelets, the coagulent heparin, blood. Blood, the most vital, the most necessary of all the organs, tissues and fluids, is coursing down the I.V. stand, entering and nourishing my daughter's body.

"Carol," I say, "you know what, the bone marrow is making platelets again and the infections are all cured. There's no more bleeding or lesions to worry about."

She nods her head in agreement, watches the last drops of the transfusion descend. "This sickie is ready to go home," she says.

Chapter 5

A hot wind blows from the desert during the three days of freedom Carol enjoys before the start of the next series of treatments; the gusts drive anxiety away, send apprehensions scudding across the Pacific Ocean which lies out of sight only a scatter of miles to the south. Carol goes buoyantly off to school, taut with excitement, an almost feverish determination apparent in her swift strides. She achieves her wish, is smuggled in to attend Senior Breakfast with Steve; signs innumerable red and white high school annuals; collects sprawling signatures and breathlessly phrased goodwill messages, vivid with sentiment, along the margins of her own annual; stands on the auditorium steps at the center of a cluster of awe-struck friends who ask tactlessly: "Carol, are you honestly here at school?" She reads the real question behind that stunned enquiry and proudly affirms her continued existence by appearing in a gay pink and green plaid dress, long-skirted and barebacked. She helps Steve while he attends Commencement rehearsals, collects his cap and gown, smiling her shimmering smile, greeting classmates, joking to everyone she meets about the absurdities of being a hospital patient in that slightly macabre manner she is acquiring.

She is seldom to be found at the house. We glimpse her rushing from place to place with the quick bright energy of a goldfinch that tries out the various twigs in a camellia bush.

34

She is a guest of the Spiri family when she attends Steve's graduation. Her own family cannot go because of the scarcity of tickets and we lose touch with her for half a day and an evening, can barely identify the flight she is making through the opacity of crowds and celebrations. The exhilaration holds, the hot desert wind is still blowing, she is laughing in the midst of her exhaustion when she re-enters the City of Hope.

We are all caught up in this mood of high exuberance. I tease Julie in the car on the way to the hospital, call her "little big mouth" because she is babbling away without restraint and the four of us unite in a spasm of laughter. We seem care-free, even well-adjusted. No raw edges are sticking out, no unevenness shows in Carol's presence.

Birdie enters the room to start the I.V. She nods briefly as Paul and Julie and I settle into chairs. She has already placed honey in the hummingbird feeder outside the room window and smiles confidentially at me, as if she were remembering our last conversation eight days ago when Carol, overcome by nausea, refused all my efforts to cheer her up. A group of high school friends appeared on the Wing, Steve among them, and Birdie whispered to me: "See, Mrs. Trautmann, she's feeling better already—here's her support. And here's that boy-girl thing, she and Steve, they've got that, and now they're learning to know each other better."

Tonight Carol decides in favor of a heparin lock, a decision which surprises Birdie. Carol, of course, is thinking of minimal trauma, not particularly of convenience. She will only need to be lanced one time; the lock will keep the vein in the wrist open for the introduction of medicines. But she will also be linked to the I.V. stand, its plastic tubes and awkward metal feet, throughout the period of treatment, being forced to wheel the apparatus along wherever she goes. The advantages of this procedure are debatable; still, Carol makes the choice.

Birdie examines Carol's wrists, avoiding the so-called "hematoma." She taps the fine veins gently. Carol's breath is coming in short bursts now, her eyes are wide and staring, she seems to have shrunk to half her normal size. No more jokes, no playfulness. Birdie finds a vein and cautiously, meticulously, tries for an injection with a slim butterfly needle. Carol shrinks even more; the vein appears to shrivel and vanish. The nurse tries again in a different spot. No luck. Birdie then asks that Julie leave the room. Surprised, Julie obliges. Carol's enormous dark eyes watch Julie's reluctant departure, then widen and stare at the nurse's capable hands.

"Carol, I got a return on this one—but it stopped. Honey, I'm so sorry," Birdie says. While I wonder whether or not Paul and I should leave, too, during the painstaking and chancy procedure, Carol clutches my arm with her one free hand and a current of tension flows between us. I stroke her softly again and again.

No one speaks. Birdie tries another time, tries once more, fails, gives it up. "Carol, I think you've lost trust in me. I'll get Mrs. De Leera to start your I.V.," she says and goes out. I feel a surge of sympathy for the baffled nurse, but stay where I am, soothing Carol until Mrs. De Leera, probing with an infinitesimal care, finally establishes the heparin lock. Long before treatment is concluded Birdie and I meet in the hallway and talk.

"I don't understand why Carol was so tense," I say. "She just tightened up all at once."

Birdie shrugs. "I don't feel bad about it," she says half-defiantly, the expression on her face unsmiling and noncommital. "As a matter of fact, you know, it happens now and again with lots of patients." Her professionalism has been ruffled, though, and I sense the pull of the finely balanced relationship between nurse and patient; the sort of challenge Carol presents because of the structure of her veins and her youthful rebelliousness. I hope Birdie will work with Carol again and I assure myself she will, although the tight look on the nurse's face does nothing to reinforce my assumption.

Julie and I come back the next morning and find Carol languid and dreamy, avoiding her breakfast. The nausea has returned. I want to maintain some confidence in nausea pills, try to regard them as preventative and salutary, but the stark truth is that these capsules do not remain in Carol's stomach any longer than the food she vomits. She keeps several square plastic containers close beside her, nibbles at an apricot, parries a slice of cantaloupe, while deliberately blocking out the aromas that stream from the warm dishes on her tray. "But unfortunately the nausea never gets any better," an aide tells me. "All of our patients have it over and over again."

Paul telephones from San Pedro. His boat, a cabin cruiser with twin engines, has developed an electrolysis problem which will keep him busy the rest of the day, perhaps longer. Listening on the portable telephone, Carol brightens, asks questions, tells her father about the brown and white cat she heard mewing outside in the shrubbery. She got out of bed, she says, and went outdoors to track down the soft plaintive sounds. "Daddy, this cat's a teen-ager, like me," she says, describing her pursuit, how she flew around the lantana bushes bare-footed.

"Keep in training, Carol, keep jogging so you can catch him," Paul advises cheerfully.

After the phone call Carol throws her head and arms forward, burying her face in the pillow on her knees. When she lifts her head again there is no trace of tears visible, only anger and frustration. "I know I'll never be able to go to Mammoth with Steve's family this summer," she says. "Why can't I just have a decent vacation like other people?"

Julie and I say nothing. We both shift our positions in the upholstered chairs.

"Can I even go to the beach, do you suppose?" she demands. "Or will I get red dots every time I walk in the sun?" We know what she is referring to, the tiny hemorrhages on her legs caused by the breakdown of the red blood cells. I listen to my own unspecific answers, the mumbling words about sun hats and beach umbrellas. Julie understands Carol's chagrin; several of her high school friends are leaving for Mexico or San Francisco or Texas. The two sisters look at each other unhappily, expressing a common bewilderment. "What kind of a crummy summer is this for our family, anyway?" Julie asks.

Carol is still at the City of Hope on Father's Day. Paul and I glance at the calendar and share some of our troubled thoughts. Only a little more than a month ago, we reflect, and specifically on Mother's Day, she was diagnosed and labelled, a mark set upon her. The bone marrow in her body has not yet made proper white cells; it may never do so. "We just have to sweat it out," Paul says grimly and then he remarks: "Don't ever celebrate these holidays, don't give me any cards or gifts ever again." I know what he is saying and I agree. There are to be no more special days for us, no festivities or celebrations from now on, only the one hammering insistent hope that Carol will survive.

I pat Blackie's rough fur and go in the living room to sprinkle fish food across the placid surface of Carol's aquarium where the tiny neon tetras and glass catfish are idly stroking the water with their delicate ribbonlike fins.

Chapter 6

I rise early. Many things need to be done and my energies are quickly consumed in small swift actions, wiping down counters, discarding empty dog food cans, scouring a skillet, unloading the dishwasher, sorting socks, collecting laundry and so on into the bathroom and after that the bedrooms. I take down my diary and vehemently report how powerful the urge to write is; I envisage the start of a short story or the completion of a poem, but end by stating that the urge to create is matched by an equally powerful urge to postpone writing. I grab a paperback copy of Tolkien's *The Fellowship of the Ring*, part one of his trilogy, and leave for the City of Hope. Perhaps Carol will let me read to her.

"Oh no, not this morning, but maybe tomorrow," she says, dodging Tolkien yet another time. It is hard to gauge her mood. She resists my suggestions to go outdoors and levels a barrage of questions at me instead. "Why can't I just start my own medicine through this heparin lock, anyway?" she asks and when she sees the paints and watercolor paper in my hands along with the paperback book, she says I am acting compulsive. She plays with words, trying to trip me up. "Don't you think I'll be alive ten years from now?" she demands. "Why are there so many older people on this Wing, why does everyone look so sick? Why don't teen-agers have leukemia?"

A minor drama develops over the morning bath. She puts it off, allows the water to cool, which subsequently infuriates the new nurse who comes in to assist Carol and keep her from getting entangled with her I.V. stand. Carol, ferociously independent, takes a cool bath without assistance from anyone. I try to pacify the distraught nurse who clearly considers Carol a "difficult" patient, and eventually the three of us achieve a state of mutual forbearance.

Carol decides to go outdoors, after all, and we sit on lawn chairs beneath dry trees that are drooping from the heat. The thermometer is near the hundred degree mark and still mounting. Carol stares at the watercolor paper, frowns, and scratches an ankle. Sitting under a tree is better than lying on a hospital bed, I reflect, reminding myself that Dr. Graham recommends more physical activity for Carol.

Can I get her to take a walk, possibly? Yes, she will walk a short distance past the petunia plantings, she promises. I notice how thin she looks, know that her weight is down to 109 pounds. The faint blue-gray tints beneath the eyes have returned and are deepening, her skin is pale, but a suggestion of pink brushes the high cheekbones, a slight tan glows on her upper arms. As she walks, crunching the gravel beneath white thong sandals, Carol wriggles her slender toes nervously. We discuss everything we can think of except leukemia.

"Carol," I say at last, "I talked to Ed Bloomfield the other evening. Remember Ed and his wife, Veronica? She's expecting a baby in December."

Carol remembers. She eyes me warily. Ed is a philosophy professor at Cerritos Community College; he is also the ebullient assistant minister at the Congregational Church not far from our house. Her memories of him, she tells me, include an autumn camping session near Redlands, cups of cold cider and apple orchards in the mountains.

"I like them both a lot," she says firmly. "Ed used to tell all the Junior High kids funny stories at camp. Really funny stories. Are you saying they want to visit me now?"

The conversation is proceeding more smoothly than I anticipated. Carol, to be sure, does not know about my first desperate phone call to Ed in May and the support he gave me then. She has never heard of the book he is mailing me, Elizabeth Kübler-Ross' *On Death and Dying*.

"As a matter of fact," I say casually to her, "Ed and Veronica would like to call on you as soon as you get back from the City of Hope."

Carol looks pleased. I brood, experience long moments of intense conflict. It is one thing to take up the role of nurse to my daughter, growing more and more aware of her changing physical and psychological symptoms. It is another matter altogether to assume the part of a spiritual or philosophical consultant. Yet that is what I am attempting to do. I mean to direct her somewhere, toward an undefined source or center. I long to succor her spirit, yearn to act and do not yearn.

For, after all, who put me in this intolerable position? I demand with resentment. Why must I guide my daughter past life's thorniest issues, answer questions I cannot resolve to my own satisfaction? Who chose me? Can I explain what ultimate reality is or what death brings in its spiny hands?

And all the other tough old chestnuts—the meaning of existence, faith, suffering, immortality. Immortality, the afterlife. Why must I grapple with such abstractions since my father wrote about them, taught and lectured about little else during his lifetime? Isn't his thinking enough, won't his faith do?

A debate rages. Someone I seldom acknowledge, the materialist within me, asks: so, what faith? Use your reason! Flesh is matter, all matter dissolves, the human destiny is destruction, nothingness. Humanity has no purpose.

I look at the delicate architecture of Carol's face, the sweeping lashes that shelter the dark eyes, the proud angle of the chin, the tapering throat that houses the soft warm voice, and my heart crumples. The materialist retreats. Another more powerful entity within me shouts *No No No No*.

"O.K.," says Carol. She gives me a smile that renders me into melting wax. "I think the Bloomfields are neat, and they had a great wedding. It was lots of fun and everybody danced afterwards, do you remember?"

I nod my head wordlessly, wondering how many ministers and chaplains have already sought out Carol. I see the leaflets on her bedside table, the paperback copies of the Bible in different versions, *The Living Bible,* a small black Catholic prayer book, Peter Marshall's prayers. Well, I reflect, if she thinks of Ed as a friend and not particularly as a minister, that should be reassuring. She might listen to him all the more.

"I wish I had known my grandfather," Carol says suddenly while I stare at her. "Something tells me he was really a strong personality." As we walk back to the entrance of Wing Five she appears to be concentrating on the image she has of my father. "How awful it must be to be blind like he was," she says with a burst of compassion before stationing the I.V. stand carefully alongside her bed.

Dr. Graham and I have another encounter in the hall when I depart. She says Carol's blood looks better, she is holding her own. They will know more at the conclusion of this present series of treatments; but Carol has not yet won remission.

I leave, wrestling with the word *remission.* No one, certainly not Dr. Graham, can realize what repercussions the term *remission* evokes for me, the ghosts that rise, the speakers I hear. "Re-mission." I test the syllables on my tongue; they possess an unmistakable ecclesiastical ring, are followed in my thought by the full-bodied phrase "remission of sins"; and, against my will, I feel myself sitting again on the hard wooden pews of a country church in the Midwest. Summer, with its bees and river banks, lies outside the heavy church doors, but I sit motionless, as if riveted to the dark oak, hearing words hurtle like angry hammers from the succession of speakers who mount the pulpit on the raised platform opposite me. It is a convocation, a church assembly of some sort, and my father and his family are honorary guests. Hand-held raffia fans are sluggishly re-circulating the summer heat. I am surrounded by attentive respectful faces, most of them furrowed and leathery tan, women wearing cotton print dresses and sturdy shoes, freckled children trying to conceal the chewing gum in their mouths. "Christ died for the remission of your sins, what will you do for Him," is the supplication that resounds from the pulpit, not once, but many times, before the final hymn is sung, five complete verses, the organ crescendos into the postlude and the crowd scatters, arms extended in fellowship, shaking hands all around.

The country church fades, I am transported to a different structure, an evangelist's tent on the outskirts of a large midwestern city, where my brother and I, uninvited and unnoticed observers, crouch in dim corners under flapping wedges of canvas. We are spies and intruders who seek entertainment, the sight of a whole congregation rolling and writhing in religious ecstasies; possibly there will be serpents and foaming at the mouth, we whisper, nudging one another. But instead the audience freezes immobilized on narrow benches, spellbound by the evangelist's ragged soaring plea. "Repent! Repent and be saved!" he beseeches them. "Sin no more, live in the hope of the remission of all your sins!"

It seems strange to me that medicine has taken over this evangelistic term which, whenever I hear it, invariably arouses a stir of uneasiness, pitting me against the uncompromising demands of the pulpit and the awesome reproaches of the revivalist.

"She has not yet won remission," I repeat to Paul. The word has exclusively medical connotations for him, I can tell. We sit on the patio together and discuss the heat and Paul's scheduled trip to Europe in July; but for the most part we muse and desperately wonder what is going on in Carol's blood.

The next day Paul and I visit the City of Hope. We interrupt Birdie in the middle of a discourse about the chemical composition of the medicines that combat leukemia. "Hi, mom and dad, guess what?" Carol says. "They're using my own blood to fight leukemia, did you know that?" Her eyes are shining. I am not certain exactly what this statement means or what Birdie has been telling her, but, listening in on the rest of the lecture I learn that the City of Hope has been using cytosine for four years now and daunomycin for one year. The latter drug has been found effective in leukemia treatments abroad, Birdie says, and the combination of the two constitutes the best chemotherapy available, at least currently. Carol hangs on to Birdie's every statement, absorbed, her confidence in the nurse apparently unshakeable; it is as if nothing had ever disturbed the composure of their relationship.

The series concludes. Carol is allowed to visit home for a few days. We pack up, overflow the suitcase and cardboard boxes with plants, magazines, yarn, vases, candy. People on the Wing say goodbye very casually. "Enjoy yourself," they exhort Carol. "Have a fine weekend."

They're all thinking the same thing, I reflect grimly, trundling the suitcase and boxes in a wheelchair to the exit. They are all quoting Dr. Graham in their minds. And I verbalize silently: "This illness isn't going to go away, Mrs. Trautmann..."

The hot rapid drive home culminates in a storm of anguish when Carol finds that a few of her house plants have died recently, whether from neglect, too little or too much watering, I cannot tell. She seems unable to tolerate any loss or change; the withering of a philodendron plant is an ominous event, over-powering her with sadness. Julie, tanned, healthy, swinging on the exercise bar over the bathroom door, tries to divert Carol's attention to the tawny cat on the front lawn, but Carol succumbs to heat and frustration. She throws herself across the water-bed, crooks Blackie in her arm and says through strangled tears; "If I die...Blackie's the only one who's going to miss me, because I brought him up from a puppy—"

Before I can cope properly with this mood Julie announces the arrival of visitors at the front door and two very old men step inside. They are churchmen, they announce soberly, representatives from an interdenominational communion on the other side of town. The wife of one of the men knew Carol years ago, taught her handicrafts during a city recreation program. It is a tenuous connection that reaches far back into the past, but that is not important, they say: what matters is the exact status of Carol's soul. The gentleman with a short brown beard stiffens on the edge of his chair. "Has she been saved?" he asks abruptly. The eyes of both men transfix me. And once more, it seems to me, I hear the rippling canvas sounds made by the evangelist's tent, the flap-flap that blurs and mingles with mid-summer haze, the hum of crickets and bees, the clamorous tones of the gesticulating revivalist.

"Carol has been baptized," I tell them. The men relax.

"She was probably baptized at the age of seven," I say weakly and then, "My father founded a religious seminary in the Midwest," I find myself adding automatically, as if this fact somehow might resolve the issue of Carol's salvation.

They do not seem to care what I say, they invite me into a circle, link hands and pray ardently for my daughter. They assure me they will continue to pray for her and for her soul.

I thank them. Their lengthy entreaties laid at the feet of an omniscient power do not resemble the prayers I myself have been composing and whispering for weeks as I work or walk or drive, the stark disjointed phrases that scorch my mind even as I think them. "God is a just God. In mercy has His throne been established," they console me, taking their leave.

"The Lord God will wipe away tears from all faces," the brown-bearded man says with fervor. "He promises justice and mercy alike to every sinner who seeks Him out and does His holy will."

These two men are the first in a succession of religious spokesmen who come to the house.

ENCOUNTER

At night I begin to waken sporadically, shaking myself out of an old recurrent dream, one which returns when I least expect it, reaching back into childhood and starting pleasantly enough, with wild raspberry bushes and beech trees, may apple and sumac massed in a thick woods just beyond the back door of my parents' home. I scout through these woods looking for something. From the particular aspect of the trees and underbrush I am able to deduce the season of the year at once and consequently can guess what I am seeking in my dream. If it is spring in all probability I peer under a shower of green leaves for trillium and dogtooth violet; if it is fall I am after dried thistle and milkweed pod. A dream of the woods can take me many different places—perhaps to random stumbling and confusion, a quagmire or to the discovery of a rare pink lady's slipper orchid. It all depends upon the path.

The woods are infiltrating my sleep now more persistently than ever before, often with an accompaniment of low thunder that rolls among branches barren of leaves and mingles with the dull monotone of hidden owls that I hear muttering in the forest depths. Sometimes I wake up from the thundery autumnal woods to find myself in the grip of a terror that subsides into chaotic thoughts and questions. What kind of night is my daughter experiencing? Is she suffering severe pain at this very moment? At other times I suddenly waken to blankness, nothing-at-all, and my mind, soft as a relaxed muscle, slowly forms the thought—see, *I am not feeling the hurt of anxiety any more!*—and immediately anguish overwhelms me.

After one such troubled night followed by a procession of slow nebulous hours at the hospital through which Carol languishes and the rest of us stagnate, I drive home, fatigued at first, but aware of an accelerating inner tempo that destroys weariness, propels me in and out of the traffic and sets me down impatiently behind my house.

There is no respite to be had here or anywhere. Sudden inexplicable energies urge me toward action. I unwind the patio hose and deluge the concrete with rapid jets of water, briskly pull weeds from the two brick planters, then seize the garden shears and begin to cut back high podocarpus shrubs. Next I cross the driveway and start up the hillside, trimming and slashing as I climb, noticing with just a fraction of my mind how overgrown the bushes seem, the shagginess of the ivy ground-cover.

Trees and flowers are in profuse bloom. I can scarcely find the brick steps that lead up the hill. The trees are bowed, almost unrecognizable in their abundance; they impinge upon each other, luxurious branches meeting to form an overhang that very closely resembles, so it strikes me, the forest canopy I once roamed beneath as a child, searching for whatever surprises the woods might provide. To be sure, of all the trees upon this slope, the sweetgum alone will turn crimson in the fall like the flaming midwestern maples I remember. The fig tree, the orange trees, avocado and apricot will remain green and immutable throughout the passing seasons.

Preoccupied, musing upon past autumns, I stumble across an invisible broken brick in the masonry steps and quickly lose my balance. Air rushes past my ears. Tree limbs are not close enough to grasp, but a flowering lantana bush helps to break my fall. I steady myself, hanging onto new shoots and crushing pungent leaves while a lizard darts over my foot like a gray arrow.

I have lost ground and must climb again. But this time the trees and tangled underbrush belong without question to the woods of my childhood and are leading me irresistibly to the back door of my parents' house. The door swings open at a touch, draws me inside to the small back hall with its high-pitched ceiling. In front of me the familiar storage cabinet for groceries, the short flight of steps that lead to the kitchen. On my right the long plunging stairs which descend into the basement. I am a child again, apprehensive, staring at the patterns of the linoleum under my tennis shoes, beige and blue squares scuffed with marks made by hard rubber heels. My knuckles tighten around the stick which I have recently picked up from half-frozen fields. Frowning, I puzzle over the linoleum squares, my nerves tensed and prickling, because someone below me in the basement is alternately shrieking and moaning. The smell of the chocolate bar in my shirt pocket sickens me.

Why is someone in the basement starting to cry? Confusion beyond in the kitchen, consternation stunning the air and the faces of the adults who materialize around me. One face is missing. Then I know the someone who cries at the foot of the cellar steps must be my aunt from the east. I am vague about the exact town and state this particular aunt lives in, but she and her husband have been spending the winter with us. Other relatives have thronged through the house, too, especially on weekends, and there has been much reminiscing about Maryland and the farm, anecdotes that sound strange to my ears, stories of carriages and horses and oil lamps. But now my quiet soft-spoken eastern aunt has just fallen down the back steps and lies in a heap moaning. Someone else, my mother, is talking at breakneck speed in shrill tones.

The adults wheel past me. Did I see what happened, do I know anything? they demand. I shake my head, no, no, yearning to run, to put the household of excited adults behind me and escape to the woods.

My mother is ill, I know this much. She is at the start of the manic phase of her cyclical illness and has been sleepless for a number of days. Above my head I can hear her voice, unusually high-keyed, answering the other adults. They plead with her while they summon an ambulance to take the aunt to the hospital. They question me further. Did she, my mother, become angry and push the aunt down the cellar stairs? I must have seen something.

I saw nothing, I tell them. A discussion rages. There is a division of thought, two viewpoints. One holds that a pregnant woman like my aunt who is carrying her first child could easily lose her balance at the top of the steps, topple over and fall. The other maintains that a frenzied woman like my mother who is ill and temporarily irresponsible could just as easily be provoked by an imagined slight, a turn of phrase wrongly interpreted, and shove the aunt backwards. The evidence is circumstantial. It is argued that my mother gardens during most of the year and is physically very strong, while the aunt is frail.

The family dilemma grows, the myth builds. When the aunt, who simply refuses to speak about the accident, loses the child she was carrying and leaves our house for good, the adults enter into a conspiracy of silence. My father happened to be absent that February day. He is never told. My mother cannot remember the event; it occupies a mysterious bleakness in her mind. A shroud of secrecy is woven that perseveres through decades and the aunt remains uncommunicative to the end of her days. If bitterness festers in anyone, it rankles in silence. But we all know the aunt never becomes pregnant again; she never carries another child....

My thoughts probe more deeply and hurtfully. Questions long unrecognized or avoided are torn out of the recesses of memory. What part did I honestly play in my aunt's life? Did I not join the adult conspiracy too, blend comfortably with the silence that obliterated her name? As soon as she left our home during that unfortunate winter, it was as if she had never been. No one spoke of her. It was easy to forget. I did not ask or wonder or think about her.

But she had existed. She loved me once. How do I know this? I cast my thought far into the past, find memories, a picture of her—a small figure unlatching windows, beckoning me outdoors into a tiny back yard. The rumble of street cars in the distance. A clump of tall sunflowers opening to the sky. The aunt's smile is sweet, directed at me. She stands before the sunflowers, the wide yellow petals framing her in a sort of halo. Suddenly she and the sunflowers are erased.

Further pictures emerge, memories even more clear-cut: the uncle from the east arriving to pay a visit, family suppers, the three brothers arguing spiritedly together. The uncle and my father talk rapidly, interrupt each other and laugh; when distance separates them again, they exchange long philosophical letters in which, I somehow intuit, the aunt is rarely mentioned. She remained invisible, she had no presence and no voice, she dwindled away and died.

A certain delicacy was at work here. Repelled by my mother's illness with its extreme moods and unpredictable behaviors, the two paternal uncles at some moment of commitment must have tacitly agreed to shield my father; their loyalty and sympathies were thoroughly aroused by the constant witnessing of his struggle with blindness, a battle he lost. They spared him whatever additional distress they could.

Who, then, spared my aunt, what solace was there for the reality of her loss?

To lose a child. The phrase leaps upon me. I reach out unsteadily and brush the rough surfaces of the wooden boundary fence, my finger tips finding crevices filled with cobwebs. I have been insensate for forty years, with no more feeling than this weather-stained cobwebbed fence. My aunt's sorrows have meant nothing to me.

To lose a child. An anguish shakes the sky and woods. The aunt's secret forgotten grief seems to mingle with my own awakened remorse. This woman we all forsook, what is to be done, how can I establish some kind of peace with her?

Silence invests the hill. Shrub and plant and tree are hushed as if stunned into soundlessness. Silence overflows from the canyons that lie to the north beyond my view and spreads like a sea ripple, meeting and embracing the quietude of my aunt's life. *Aunt Nan.* These two syllables are wrenched out of me; they drop like stones into a pond and rest expectantly under water, soon to be overlaid by sifting mud and more silence.

Silence breeds fear, unreasoning raw fear, claws that tear at the mind. *Aunt Nan, wherever she is, might want my child now. Because I, too, abandoned her, I may now be compelled to suffer as she did, learn what she learned.* A great iron scale balances above me; I can sense the swing of it, back and forth, unsettling the air.

Surely there is a way. I will exonerate myself, confront my aunt, explain how young and ignorant I was in those days. She will forgive me. She will require nothing from me. But how does anyone make explanations to the dead? What kind of communication? How?

I look about me. Everywhere in the warp and woof of the hillside, fresh contours, flourishing growth, newness, rampant life. No hint of death. The fig tree bears fruit; the orange trees are laden with both fruit and flowers. Slim unripe avocados droop like jewels among shiny leaves. One shrub alone, the pomegranate, can be associated with death since, according to Western mythology, it produced the food Persephone ate before her release from Hades.

A single pomegranate bush glitters before me now, covered with large red-orange blossoms. Very well, *durch die Blume*, then, *through the flower*. I gather flowers until my arms enfold a bonfire of orange petals and yellow stamens. What is it I expect to happen, though? I stand uncertainly, under the weight of brilliant blossoms, straining every sense. I would like a sign, or a message, some indication that the long forgotten aunt knows of my need and responds. I wait. Long minutes go by. The hill stays quiet and motionless. But the quality of the silence has changed and my nerves, which remain taut as before, are no longer raw with fear. The claws have receded.

Perhaps there have been too many years of silence, I tell myself, and Aunt Nan may have lost the will to communicate with the living; or she may be waiting for another more propitious moment. Or perhaps other ways to reach the dead exist; I should be patient and hope to discover them.

I can indicate a sign, though, even if my aunt cannot. All over the world, I reflect, people leave offerings of candles, incense, coins, on every kind of altar. I will leave my offering here. I place the pomegranate blooms on the ground and around their fiery core I erect a wide border of ripe and unripe fruit.

I select the finest of the ginger lilies, golden lantana and rose hibiscus, wreathing the whole with ivy leaves the color of deep sea water and I carry the cluster down from the hill into the house. I think of my aunt as I go, but I think of my mother also, the careful gardener who worked the earth's rich soil with tenderness and patience during the best days of her life. I set the flowers and ivy within the largest vase I can find, in memory of my mother, to honor her.

Chapter 7

As the temperature readings soar higher, the small air conditioning unit anchored in the corner of Carol's bedroom collapses. "What are we going to do now?" I expostulate to Paul. "The heat is simply unbearable. Can the house be air-conditioned, do you think?"

"Well, there are difficulties," he answers, going on to elaborate, but the explanations only cause me to lose my temper. "It is 105 degrees!" I shout at him. "One hundred and five! Look at us, look at Carol, we are reduced to tallow. Or maybe it's ash. And, by the way, do you know what she did yesterday?"

"No," he replies uneasily, "but please calm down."

"She got out our old medical encyclopedia, it has four volumes, you know, and it's really old, this edition was published the year she was born, 1956," I narrate. Paul looks at me.

"Well, there are lesions like little buds forming on the side of her tongue and she's gargling with salt water and saying to me, 'Mother, see, I am trying to take care of myself...'" and then she takes down the medical books and begins to read, I can't stop her, and all at once she says 'Mother, if I have Hodgkin's disease, I'll kill myself.'"

Paul catches his breath. "Can't you hide that encyclopedia somewhere?" he asks.

"Oh yes, sure," I cry. "Fine, after she's already read the articles on cancer, blood disease, leukemia and God knows what else. And the difference between chronic and acute leukemia, do you know what she read, what she believes?"

Paul watches me.

"The article in that encyclopedia says that chronic leukemia requires treatment for a number of years, but acute leukemia does not. Do you know how she interprets this?" I cannot keep the tears back. "She thinks... she'll be cured soon." I break down and wail, the sounds I utter are unrecognizable, they bruise my own ears.

Paul makes an unsteady effort to console me. He suggests activities, urging that I focus on hiking or swimming. "Or keep busy in women's groups," he says. "What about beginning some night school classes again? Please, try not to take the frustrations out on me."

"All right," I say, now knowing what it is I am agreeing to. "I'll do better."

For solace Paul turns to his shop. I go to my diary and write like an automaton without interest or expectations, until I find the pain easing slightly and discover words of encouragement filling up the pages. "I can at least do this much," my diary counsels. "I can form words, pin down fear and hope on paper. Words are builders, they construct. And if the inexplicable enters my life, as it has, I can surely begin to realize that others feel the same way I do. Pain is everywhere, a commonality linking us to one another, and in this inter-relatedness of all life I shall certainly find strength... and if I tell myself these things often enough," my diary concludes, I believe I will believe them."

Words help, talk helps, friends sustain, but at the same time disquieting emotions gravitate to the surface where I must examine them: resentment for my husband's mobility, so much greater than mine, the fact that he can leave frequently for San Pedro to work on his boat, saying "we'll take Carol on short boat trips soon" or depart for other states and foreign countries; an ever-deepening lethargy that on some days unites with an unfathomed fear and almost immobilizes me; a sense of floundering; a lurking fatalism that I resist as much as possible, relating it to a negation of free will and the cancellation of choices. This whole complex of emotions simply evaporates whenever I confront the reality that is molding my inner life, the recumbent figure on the water-bed who clutches her black spaniel tightly while she studies the calendar with eager questioning eyes.

I put down the diary to pick gardenias from the bush under the kitchen window and float the flowers in round clear bowls of water, because Ed and Veronica are coming over.

They both greet Carol and Julie and me as if a handful of days, not two years, have passed since the five of us met together. "What beautiful girls you have," Ed says in an aside to me; he is including Amy also in this remark, he says with a smile, and a warm glow settles over the room while we reminisce about camping and youth groups. He mentions picnics, car pools and the inexhaustible varieties of tuna-fish sandwiches. We all laugh.

Veronica, whose long hair is twisted and coiled at the nape of her neck, is a nurse of considerable experience; she knows a number of women who have taken their training at the City of Hope. "Carol, when did you first realize you were ill?" she asks.

Carol answers a little doubtfully, saying the symptoms were vague, but changes were occurring, she just wasn't feeling right. "I talked to Les, one of my girl friends," she admits shyly. "It was while we were at the beach during Easter vacation. I said 'Les, don't tell anybody, but I think I've got cancer or something else awful'...I'd been worrying a lot," she confesses, turning her glance away from mine to scrutinize a corner of the living room rug.

"And what did the doctor tell you?" Ed asks carefully. Carol's reply is clear and matter-of-fact, devoid of gloom, without a single prediction or statistic. There is an immediate and indefinable relaxation of tension, a pause, during which everyone seems to be deliberating.

"What do you want to study, Carol? What do you want to do with your life?" Ed says. With a slight wrench I realize no one has asked Carol that question since her diagnosis.

"Why, I want to study medicine," she says calmly. Her eyes lock with mine. I attempt to minimize my alarm by talking about high school and the award in advanced foods she has just won. "But I really do want to study medicine," she says considering me gravely.

The conversation shifts to colleges, those nearby, especially the community colleges: Cerritos, Rio Hondo, Mount San Antonio, the names rolling off our tongues like a Spanish litany. Ed off-handedly mentions an Arab student, a young man interested in philosophy, who has chosen to study in California because he receives such excellent treatment for his leukemia here. Carol absorbs this bit of news with obvious appreciation.

We are living in Artesia now, Ed and Veronica remark, saying goodbye; and they ask us to call them any time, any time at all. Down at the curb I give them a copy of a poem of mine which has recently appeared in a feminist magazine. For a few minutes we chat about Tolkien and fantasy.

After their visit I feel refreshed; and relieved, also, as if Ed and Veronica comprise a sort of spiritual reservoir—genuine, trustworthy, responsive—that is available to Carol and me both.

I find Carol in front of a full-length mirror trying on a yellow wrap-around dress she has just finished sewing. With pins in her mouth she tells me how much she likes Ed and Veronica and asks: "But how come you jumped so high when I said I wanted to study medicine?"

"Oh, I don't know," I reply. "I suppose I thought you hadn't decided on a career yet."

"But I'm really keen about chemistry, Mom," she says. "Besides I got an A in it." She hugs me. "Please don't call the hospital, promise?" she asks. "Don't tell Dr. Graham about the sores on my tongue, O.K.? I'm getting a blood check tomorrow anyhow."

Startled, I agree.

Carol adjusts the yellow print dress in a matter of minutes and is ready to go out with Steve. Just before he arrives she places an enormous gum-ball in her mouth, positions it carefully at one side where it causes a great bump to protrude. "Thee, Thteve, my tongue ith tho thwollen," she announces to her startled boy friend. His panic-stricken reaction delights her.

Oh well, I sigh to myself, another practical joke, she must be feeling better, anyway.

The following morning Dr. Graham tells us that the antibiotics are causing the lesions to form on Carol's tongue. She can go back home, take good care of herself, and return in five days for more treatment. The doctor mentions some other matters that are concerning her—the enovid, which should be more effective in preventing hemorrhage than it actually is, the necessity of arranging for Carol to have a period; young girls with leukemia encounter quite special problems, she hints. I listen, feel a growing sense of helplessness invade me.

At the house again, Julie is bursting with good news. She is planning a jaunt to Oceanside with friends, will borrow a wet suit from someone and try skin diving. Carol receives this information without comment. Later, I discover her in the tub, ringed by soapy water, crying softly into the soap bubbles.

I step back into the shadows, lean against the closed hallway cupboard for support. What is it like to be Carol? I ask myself. Can I enter that sensitivity for a while, experience its painful wonderment?

Very well, I shall be Carol.

See, I am out of range now, removed from the inquisitiveness of both doctor and parent. I can conduct a cautious search of my own body, face the relentless self-questioning: what does this minute scratch mean, what will it lead to? How much longer will my gums bleed? Why does the skin around my ankles itch and flake?

To be Carol, equably discussing the future, when there

may never be any. To talk about high school graduation and college and then stop talking all at once, because the truth is, whenever I enter a room crowded with human beings, relatives, friends, or students, I take my life in my hands, I risk a death.

To be Carol is to watch the invisible at work, to be aware of the subtle manifestations of change others are not perceiving; to live in an aureole observing the new bright edges that suddenly illuminate all the objects of the earth; to see the familiar and the loved invested with light. The glance directed by my eyes is a caress, stroking each remembered person and possession, each mark of the landscape, with a desperate tenderness. My hands shake as they gently brush the pages of an old fairytale book I have cherished for years, see, I recall every single picture and story; my fingers enfold a round painted stone, loving its smooth perfection; the raffia heart tied with a pink ribbon, the fragments of petrified wood from New Mexico, the blue and white balloons, the red silk rose, see, I remember, I love and treasure everything I touch. And no one is watching, I will close my eyes and let the tears stream freely, wherever they will: to lose all this and more, to leave, to part, to have the fibers of my being torn...

I separate myself from Carol, emerge from an enchantment, but only partially, because when she walks down the hall toward the living room, her hair flowing in broad corn-colored waves, I seem to be watching Persephone. "My daughter, my daughter," I say under my breath, sinking deep into her thought again.

She brings me back to the present, kisses me goodbye. She is off on a drive with high-school companions, a very modern young woman holding a bottle of ice water and a sack of potato chips; but then, I notice, like the Hesperides, the daughters of Hesperus who preside over the mystic gardens at the rim of the world, she is carrying some golden apples in her arms, too.

Chapter 8

Carol sleeps late the following morning and when I open her door Blackie catapults across the room and bites me on the stomach. His barking awakens her. She sees my torn blouse and at once begins to spank the dog with a rolled up newspaper.

"Bad dog, Blackie!" she cries. "You irritating animal! Mom, did he hurt you?"

"No, no, not a bit," I say. "Blackie just thinks he's a dragon and you're the sleeping princess he's supposed to protect. Inside that fuzzy head of his a lot of fairy stories are rattling around."

Carol raps the newspaper across the quivering black rump again. "Some dragon," she says without smiling, but Blackie, undeterred, assumes his stance alongside the bed, legs apart, nose raised high, fracturing the air with his nervous bark.

"I came in to show you these," I say and pass several square-cut samples of green carpeting above the dog's agitated head. "The painter has already been here earlier this morning to look at the living room."

"But why didn't you wake me?" she protests, wrinkling her forehead in an effort to concentrate on the swatches. I merely shrug as I glance around the room, approving its fresh colors, the orange and green, yellow and brown of the flowered bedspread and curtains, Carol's recent selections, chosen in between bouts of chemotherapy.

"Brighten the place up for us, will you, Carol?" Paul and I continue to urge casually, turning the task of redecorating the living room over to her and Julie as if it were an after-thought, not a project meant to keep both daughters busy.

"Hey, Carol!" Paul calls from the back yard. "Come out here, won't you? I need your advice." Carol responds by throwing on a robe and running. She grabs a banana in her quick transit through the kitchen.

Paul, perspiring, breathing deeply, stands with one foot resting on a shovel, triangles of red adobe soil heaped to the left and right. The narrow strip of ground that lies next to the garage and outside his shop door is rapidly becoming an empty clay pit.

"But daddy," Carol exclaims, "do you just have to dig up the whole back yard today?"

"Why certainly, Carol. I've got to put a sprinkler system in here first," he says, "and then you can have a go at it."

"Me, daddy?" she asks, bewildered.

"Sure, honey," he says. "You can plant a garden, grow anything you want to." He beams, contemplating this new project for her. "What's your pleasure, Carol, flowers or how about radishes and tomatoes, maybe?"

His shop radio is turned on and before Carol can make a suggestion the tense voice of a news commentator shrills out the stock market report and the weather, pauses, then announces the death of a famous football coach who, having just observed his fiftieth birthday, but afflicted with many ailments including a weak heart and kidney complications "died late last night...only two years after he was discovered to be suffering from acute leukemia..."

Paul and I stare at each other. Carol sits down abruptly on a child's redwood bench that is positioned against the garage wall. "I wonder if he was ever treated at the City of Hope," she says.

"Look, he was a very sick man. He had all sorts of things wrong with him, and he wasn't young to begin with," Paul starts to explain. He is filling the silence with words. Carol shakes her head up and down slowly, as if agreeing, but her thoughts no longer seem directed toward the back yard or the future garden or us.

"Daddy, do you want me to help with the shovel?" she asks after a while and, being reassured that her effort is not needed at this point, she quietly goes back into the house. I follow her. She gets out the sun lamp, puts on a halter top and shorts and adjusts dark glasses over her eyes.

"Here, Carol, use these please," I say, giving her two cotton pads to place under the tinted lenses. She takes them absentmindedly.

"Kim was a patient at the City of Hope just before she died." It is a statement, a fact we are both remembering, and Carol continues, as if picking up the thread of my own thought. "...She was always so small and pretty. She used to come over and play on the hill sometimes with Amy and Julie and me, but I was the one who knew her best. We both loved horses. And later on Kim really learned how to ride and won lots of ribbons. she was really good and had her own horse, besides."

And Kim died only last January, I think, my mind pacing with Carol's. She died of a rare bone disease, she was in chemotherapy, too, how much did her treatment resemble the treatment for myeloblastic leukemia? And what can I do to divert these thoughts, anyhow?

Carol lies beneath the sun lamp, its rays casting a strong blue-white circle upon her legs. "Don't stay too long under that," I warn unnecessarily, conscious of the kitchen timer ticking away noisily at her elbow. I proceed into the yellow bedroom and adjust the curtains, pulling on the cords and thinking about Kim and the boy who died in room 531 at the City of Hope; and six months ago before all this began, someone else Carol knew died unexpectedly, Joe what-was-his name? I frown, recalling the night she attended the rosary held for him, picturing her with my black lace handkerchief pinned over her blond hair. And does one death lead to another, a sort of psychic chain reaction, can Carol be thinking as morbidly and illogically as I am just now?

A small brown leather-bound book I have never seen before lies on her dresser. I take it up wonderingly. It is a prayer book. A flat black ribbon uncurls from the pages assigned to prayers for those seriously ill. I open the book, detect a few faint pencil underlinings and read: "...*preserve this suffering servant from the devil's temptations, pity the hopelessness of his sins, restore him to health if Thou wilt.*"

What is this? I read further: "*Deliver him from evil and mischief and sin, from the wrath of everlasting damnation.*"

Carol has been reading this? I drop onto the waterbed. Under the impact of my body the loose plastic mattress gives a loud splashing response, several reverberations that instantly remind me of flopping canvas. Here he is again, the tent evangelist of my childhood, eloquent and persuasive, his thunderous words and heavy thought invading the still bedroom: sin, guilt, the hopeless human condition.

"*Be not angry with me forever*" is the last line my astonished eyes take in from the open pages. And who could be angry with Carol forever?

Chapter 9

Carol walks into her room and finds me puzzling over the brown prayer book. "Who in the world gave you this?" I ask at once.

"Oh, a friend," she says. Her mouth firms. She does not intend to tell me more.

"Well, yes, perhaps," I say. It is not an auspicious phrasing, so I start over again. "Carol. These prayers. Don't you think they sound, well, harsh?"

She is listening to me.

"I want you to understand. When you used to attend Sunday school or when you and I went to church together, I'm certain you never heard about a god who punishes people forever."

She smiles at me. "The mean-old-man-god?" She asks lightly. Her expression changes, the smile departs. "On Monday night," she says slowly, "I went to a party."

"Yes, I know you did."

"People kept coming up to me and asking how I feel. They were saying 'Gosh, Carol, you look great.' That's what most of them said but there were others, mom, some I didn't know very well—" The dark eyes are fixed on me, they are my own eyes, a blend of green and brown, a true hazel stare, uncompromising, steady. "These people look at me as if I were dying, mother."

I try to counter this, I say quickly, "Carol, we are all dying, each one of us, every single day."

"Yes, of course," she says, "but some of us are dying more rapidly than others. I am. I am dying faster than you or anyone else I know."

A sob wrenches my throat. "You are going to get well!" I shout. "You can recover from this," I say more calmly. "You can. You will." I pick up the brown book, riffle its pages. "Whatever you read," I say, "please choose, be more selective. Is it all right if I make a suggestion?"

"Sure, if you want to."

I ponder, and then leave the room for a few minutes, returning with an armful of books. "Suppose I hang onto that little prayer book," I suggest, "and you keep these in exchange."

Carol silently agrees.

"Do you promise to really look at them?"

Carol agrees again.

"Good. Well, then, here are the Psalms, an edition my mother gave me." I hand her the thin white volume. "And here's a small book of rosaries, prayers to Mary. I had a cousin once," I reflect, "though it seems like a thousand years ago, who wanted to become a Carmelite nun, and she came to live with us for a time. She left me this."

Carol examines the book of rosaries.

"And now these are some things your grandfather wrote. The encyclopedia has an article in it written by him." I place the thick volume on the dresser and stack four more books on top of it. I lay one final item in Carol's hand, a round card printed in red and blue letters. "A passage-finder," I explain. "Choose your topic, move the wheel, the arrow points to different verses in the Bible."

"What to read," Carol enunciates precisely, "when you are lonely, when you are in doubt, when you are angry, when you are sick...well, yes. I guess I will." She stares as if hypnotized by the cardboard circle.

"Mother, I'm afraid." She begins to speak hurriedly, unburdening herself. "I'm afraid I have the fast-moving kind of leukemia, like the Elwood's granddaughter, who died in fifteen hours, I think it was, and I don't know how much time I have left either, whether it's minutes or hours or months or what."

I stroke her hair, the curve of her arm. "No one knows how much time is left," I manage to say. For a very long moment we stand side by side, Carol downcast, shuttered into her private despair, I caressing her with the lightest touch my fingers can trace.

"Once when I thought I had cancer," I begin, "I was so frightened, I remember how hard everything seemed to..." But Carol's startled eyes are betraying shock.

"Listen, dear," I say hastily. "We are all in this together, we are with you every single minute. You are never, never just by yourself. Believe me. And believe that you're going to get well. Because we know that you will."

Carol gives me a swift comprehensive hug. She brightens. The room seems to pulsate with light and vitality. "I'm so lucky," she says, shaping one of her reckless non-sequiturs. "My mother is a writer. And my father is a businessman." She kisses me. "You know what I plan to do now? I'm going outdoors to ask daddy if I can have another pet."

She laughs at the expression on my face. "Don't worry, mom, it's okay. I just want the raccoon I saw last night climbing the silk oak tree in the dark. I could barely make out its white mask and bushy tail. Wouldn't it be great to own a raccoon?"

She kisses me a second time, dashes off breathlessly to tease her father into capturing the raccoon, resilient and happy, determined that no shadow will obscure the world she loves. For three days she does not mention the City of Hope. Carol, Debbie and Les, a high school triumvirate first put together in seventh grade and by now welded into permanency, go shopping for records and dress material. I hear the cacophony of rock music, observe folds of brown and white cloth come into the house, a yard of cotton festive with lemons and green leaves that is quickly sewn into shorts. I am introduced to two hermit crabs and a turtle. Carol's lightheartedness holds. Individual notes of her clear laughter reach me occasionally; as if drifting through a hedge they detach themselves and incise an indelible musical notation on the tablet of my mind.

The day before she is expected to return to the hospital a cold finger of dread flickers for a moment across her happiness. "When I go back," she says, helping me hose off the rusty barbecue grill on the patio, "if they want me to take another bone marrow test, I'm not going to let them do it."

"Don't think about that," I say, sensitive to her reactions and hating the pain and inconvenience of the bone marrow tests also. "Face whatever comes up today. Don't deal with tomorrow yet. For now, see if you can find any charcoal, please."

That evening Carol and Paul watch one of the several Watergate exposés being shown on television. "Daddy, is this as bad as the Teapot Dome scandal?" Carol asks, trying to fit Watergate into her high school government courses. But Paul is so engrossed he only mutters a distracted "...ummm, probably" and Carol, drowsing, falls asleep on the couch beside her father. It is a fitful nap. She wakens, goes into the kitchen and calls me.

"What's the matter, Carol?" I trail her around the corner away from the noise of the television set.

"Mother, you know what, I still bruise like a peach," she says, showing me a discoloration on her right leg. "I think I might need another transfusion again soon."

There is something she wants from me. "Could I wear a couple of your elastic hose for a while? My legs ache."

"Of course." I rummage through dresser drawers and find two tight elastic stockings. She puts them on eagerly. Before long she is finished with Watergate, yawning into the folds of her robe, ready to go to bed. For a brief instant my arms surround her tremulously, with an infinite caution, because she rests inside my awkward embrace unaware that I am shielding a newborn child—my second daughter, endearing, tenacious, whose small arms clasp my neck tightly, whose shock of dark hair fills my mouth and blocks out the tiny narrow face that is rosy with strawberry marks, the deep pink splotches which the doctor assures me will vanish, perhaps in seven more days.

I go to bed, too. The air in the dimly lighted back bedroom seems stifling. Suddenly I can hear my own blood coursing through its many channels, feel the distention of the veins in both legs like whipcords that pulse and beat. I know what varicose bruises are smudging my own body and do not need to locate them, their mauve networks, their ripe strawberry stains.

Minutes later when Paul retires and Carol's voice calls across the darkness "Goodnight, daddy; goodnight mother" I try to answer, murmur indistinctly and give myself over to tears.

Morning arrives streaked with fog and I find Carol leaning out an open window watching the birds on the lawn. "Just sneaking the birdies a few tidbits," she says, gesturing at the flat wooden tray on the window ledge that is half-filled with birdseed. She cocks her head. "Will you listen, he's come back. It's the first time I've heard him this summer." She is talking about the mockingbird and pointing into the gray-green center of the tasselled bottlebrush tree. The tones pouring from the shaking leaves are operatic, unmistakably those of a mockingbird.

"Show-off, isn't he?" she says. I realize that Blackie, motionless for once, is draped over her arm and the gray cat named Mousey is purring on a pillow only inches away from the dog's drooping tail.

"You know what, Carol, you remind me of someone," I say but she is half out the window again and cannot hear me. It doesn't matter, I muse, she seldom browses in old art books and has probably never seen a photograph of "the lady of the beasts."

"This is the second summer for the mockingbird," Carol says, still watching the tremor in the depths of the bottlebrush tree. She meticulously arranges a few large gray and white striped seeds in a neat circle on the feeding tray. "Do you think he'll be coming back here again next year?"

Chapter 10

It is the same room as last time. The same medical opinion, too. "She is holding her own." Dr. Graham smiles encouragingly at Carol, then talks to me privately and says the blood is not doing what it should. She is not responding to the daunomycin. At the conclusion of the next series following this one, that is, the fifth series, a new treatment will be attempted. A different chemotherapy. We will not tell Carol, of course, not yet.

I return to the hospital room bone-chilled, a physical condition I recognize, a sensation like stepping into a gravel pit, the sudden contact with cold water that numbs the feet and ankles and sets an iciness spiraling upward through the viscera. Many years ago during warm summers I used to swim occasionally in gravel pits, although they were off limits for the public; and though people warned they had no bottom, a rock thrown into them would sink endlessly, a swimmer might drown. In those days I was young and impatient and relished a challenge. How different it is now during this summer of hypnotic rhythms and blazing heat! I am a slow-paced underwater swimmer suspended within bottomless channels washed by successive streams from an invisible gravel pit; and I am truly terrified.

Carol is obviously feeling neglected. Her father has left for Europe, Julie for Oceanside. Most of her friends are settling down on one California beach or another. So she's alone,

I reflect. Everyone loves Carol, but wants to forget the leukemia for a while.

Carol frets, examines the bruises on her thighs, makes new discoveries. "Just look at these red dots," she says. "They're not even red any more; they're turning gray and getting larger, too. What does that mean, lack of platelets, or something else?"

It is frightening to watch the whole I.V. ritual even if Birdie is administering the medication and continues to be cheerful and supportive. My morale plummets. Desperate questions pour in from the frigid depths I flounder through. I cannot escape them. Where are the pain, the nausea, stress, tedium and suspense all leading? Where are Carol and I going?

I return to an empty house in Whittier. Trying to exorcise the fear that numbs me, I roll down my car window and cry to the passing traffic: "She will respond, she'll get well, she will, you'll see!" Uncaring, the freeway drivers and their cars melt into a continuum of gray streaks.

As if waiting for me, her empty green robe sways from a wire hanger above the hall door. Unexpected bursts of wind shake the garment, endowing it with motion. I hide my face in the soft quilted fabric; I can smell cologne, traces of fragrant powder. The pale green folds contain only an illusion of life; the sleeves hang straight and flat, the buttons lie cold against my cheek.

What shall I do? I shout at the echoing house, the swinging robe. What do you want me to do? Blackie comes running down a hallway that suddenly looms labyrinthine and secretive. He cannot comfort me very much; his post remains alongside the waterbed where he returns snuffling to take up guard duty again.

She has left a large library book on the coffee table in the living room, *Birds and Mammals of North America*. I open its pages, pat the shiny pictures of robins and otters. This very morning at the City of Hope Carol, restive and irritable, would not allow me to touch her, and so now I stroke the photographs in her library book instead, soothingly, dreaming the moments away.

I must leave this deserted house. As the thought forms, my feet spurt across the room, down the brick porch. They accelerate until I am almost racing when I reach the Lil Ol Taco Maker's Drive-In on Whittier Boulevard. I wait at the curb for my order of tacos to be filled. Automobiles drift past, time idles.

All at once I crumple and clutch the telephone pole that slants skyward beside me. The wood splinters, fragments pierce the tender flesh under my nails, but I am sobbing and do not care. I speak to the wooden pole that was once a tree. I recite prayers, Protestant, Catholic, Jewish phrases; the names of God in every tradition and language that comes to mind; invocations to the saints and to the evangelists, Matthew, Mark, Luke and John—but I cannot remember the names of all the disciples.

"Please excuse me." An old man carrying tortillas steps up to the curb. "Madam, do you need any help?"

"Oh, no, certainly not," I assure him. I claim my tacos and run.

At home the telephone rings. Marlene Spiri calls about the trip to Mammoth, which would include, she says, five days in the mountains, plenty of rest for Carol, a comfortable cabin, breath-taking views of forests and lakes. Surely Carol can go?

"This is confidential, but there may be a change in treatment soon," I say, my voice wobbly. "Dr. Graham reports she isn't responding to the daunomycin."

"Oh, but she will." Marlene's confidence acts like a restorative and in spite of my terrors I tell her," Yes, I'm certain Carol will be able to go to the mountains..."

Others call: neighbors, church members, nursery school teachers who remember Carol, friends that used to assist me when I led a Girl Scout troop, women activists, who are organizing a hot line for rape victims. "Mary, please come and visit us," they say. "Let us know when you are available. We want to help." Their compassion opens up a warm countercurrent within the chill watery spirals of the gravel pit.

A letter addressed to me arrives from the head of the Blood Replacement Program at the City of Hope. Carol's transfusions are withdrawing a good many pints of blood from the reserves and I am being asked to replenish the supply. None of us has thought much about the source of the blood that descends with such exasperating slowness from the plastic packets strung on the I.V. stands. People donate blood, I realize, only they can give this gift; and it is to people that I must turn now.

I galvanize a network of human beings, ministers, secretaries, next-door neighbors, Debbie, Les, Carol's club members, and finally, Milwaukee. "Sure, of course," my sister and oldest daughter tell me. "We'll be glad to donate blood in Carol's name. How is she?"

I do not know how to reply. The simple question is unanswerable and my dry throat rasps to find an appropriate response.

The next day a neighbor drives to Duarte with me. At the sight of Carol in a hospital bed, Joyce falters and her British accent broadens, but she extends the card and the beribboned package she is carrying with characteristic cheerfulness. "You've got the best room in the house, you know that, don't you, love?" she says lightly.

We have come at an emotionally charged moment. Steve Spiri, arms folded over his chest, stands frowning into a bouquet of pink rosebuds. Carol is scowling at the square of lemon jello on her tray. When I mention the letter from the blood bank and the request for donors, Carol's anger erupts.

"Mother!" she fumes. "Don't you dare phone my friends and ask for blood! Don't you dare call up my friends, ever!" Her fist pounds for emphasis, the jello vibrates.

"But Carol—" I protest and stop, alarmed by the storminess of her expression.

"I'm a big girl now," she insists.

Someone changes the subject. Joyce tells a funny story and soon Carol and Steve are both laughing. The repartee heightens.

Dinner trays arrive in the room. Carol waves goodby to us over the flower vases, the freshly opened napkins and the inquiring heads of the hospital aides.

CALICO

She comes to us near Halloween under the sign of Scorpio which is Carol's sign, too: Calico, the long-haired tortoise-shell cat, appropriately endowed with masses of orange and brown-black fur and with large copper eyes. She is everyone's cat at first, does not become Carol's cat for years.

Assuming her obvious shyness masks a willingness to please, I am confident the Halloween cat will tolerate children, that her temperament will adjust nicely to those young temperaments in our own household belonging to Amy, Carol and Julie. This is what I tell Paul; and, half-enchanted by the copper-moon eyes, we take her from the pet store and bring her to the house where she is smothered with affection, teased and stroked and fed too much milk. Paul is not certain he likes Calico. She seems skittish to him. And almost at once my own opinion of the tortoise-shell undergoes revision, because her shyness conceals both introversion and a fierce independence. The superficial kittenish behavior soon matures into adulthood; she rapidly by-passes adolescence and meets and mates with a gray tomcat on the hill and is ready to present us with kittens.

I have theories about pets. They are useful instructors in the dramas of life, I relate to my husband, and undoubtedly the reason this cat has come to us at all is to initiate our daughters to the realities of motherhood. The cycles and tribulations of animals hold invaluable meanings for children, I say. Calico is meant to demonstrate birth, just as our first household pet of any size and significance, the enormous white duck named Quack who used to frequent the hillside behind the house, most certainly enacted the reality of death for our children's edification.

Paul points out that Quack did not die naturally but was waylaid and slaughtered by a predatory opposum; neither he nor I have been able to explain such a misfortune or the rationale of loss adequately to our three daughters who question us almost daily about Quack's unexpected demise. Amy, Carol and Julie merely know that their former pet's remains now lie buried on the hilltop close to the chain link fence where the restive Quack, much too plump and clumsy for flying, once paced back and forth raising great snowy wings in hapless appeals to the air. He and his snakelike neck, the haughty postures, ill temper and angry beak are suddenly gone, bones and plumage laid in the ground beside the small pets that preceded him—the parakeet, the chameleon, the fish. A sequence is established, I remark; the tortoise-shell cat must be entering our lives to distract us from Quack's dying and preoccupy three children with the fascinations of multiple birth.

The theory seems plausible but what I cannot account for is my own antipathy to Calico's presence in the house. There is an eerie quality about her. She sulks. Her lack of sociability frustrates me. I am unable to suppress a feeling of revulsion when I see her lurking in the corners like a nervous shadow. She shrinks from my proffered affection, is always springing just out of range, as if the touch of my hand would scorch her. Calico's fidgety manners make me more and more uncomfortable; I frequently consign her to the outside, so that slowly, imperceptibly, she changes from a house cat to an outdoors cat.

"It's not because of your pregnancy," I tell Calico, dislodging her from the laundry room and shooing her across the patio, "because, honestly, I'm with you there, I understand pregnancy. No," I say, "it's your attitude. You're too unsociable, too wild." As she vanishes into the shrubbery I feel an illogical yearning to go with her in her wanderings, visit her haunts, the avocado branch where she likes to crouch, the roof shingles where she suns herself.

Calico is still domesticated in part. She appears regularly for meals, she eats voraciously without becoming huge, stays indoors for tidbits, catnip and attentions from her three young admirers, but returns as soon as possible to the comforts of the hillside where she and the gray tom she has taken up with construct a home deep in the ivy and ginger lily stalks. Paul says she is manifesting a peculiarly female trait, the "nesting instinct."

"Maybe, that lair of hers certainly looks like a bird's nest," I say. "She has the strangest habits, perhaps she's the Cheshire Cat, come back from Wonderland." Paul says he has never read *Alice*, but Calico is an odd one, all right. And then suddenly on a sunny April afternoon in between plates of mackerel and saucers of milk, Calico disappears.

The gray tomcat acts distracted, confused. Amy, Carol and Julie pool their observations and thoughts, decide that Calico has left the slope and built a new retreat, a better nest, possibly at the edge of the swamp in Sycamore Canyon. The canyon lies some distance beyond the crest of the hill. Searching it would involve a very long hike, but before I am dragooned into leading a scouting expedition, Calico displays herself walking proudly along the top of the pink brick wall in the back yard. She preens and poses, self-assured, her particolored body noticeably flattened.

"Daddy! Mother!" the three daughters shriek. "Calico has had her babies! Where are they, where are they?" The pursuit is on. Calico stops her posturing. She senses at once that her three friends are after the new-born kittens. She will not be pinned down or coaxed into making revelations. She becomes a shifting shadow, more mobile than ever, a fluid streak of orange and black fur.

She lures her rapt followers, takes them on travels around the neighborhood from one back yard to another, apricot tree to weed patch, fence to geranium border. She lopes away, returns, mews, begs for food, vanishes as soon as she is fed, a game that contunues for seven whole days, a week during which no one glimpses a single kitten. "But why don't we stop running after her?" someone suggests. "Let's just sit in the living room and watch, find out where it is she's really going every day. Maybe the kittens aren't even hidden outdoors or on the hill at all."

And they aren't. We discover them lying only a few feet away, huddled inside the hollow back of the old Hi Fi cabinet, resting on a cache of torn paper and yarn and other oddments

Calico has assembled to accommodate the four squirming sightless creatures she has borne. We are awed, the children especially so, captivated by Calico's tactics and resourcefulness. No one wants to disturb her new nest.

But eventually the mother and four offspring emerge from the shelter of the Hi Fi, and each daughter adopts one gray and white female for her own. The only unclaimed kitten is a yellow striped male, instantly dubbed Blondie, who becomes a floater, foot-loose and pampered and a little vain. The three gray and white pets are christened with unremarkable diminutives, Mousey, Milky, Fuzzy, and during the weeks that follow all four kittens play together indefatigably, their antics and clowning very much appreciated by everyone except Calico who simply exhibits a mild tolerance or scorn and refuses to stay grounded in maternity for long. She stops nursing, is spayed, and avoids the gray tom. Calico leaves the kittens to us and goes off on frequent nocturnal journeys, visits other streets and alleys and orchards.

"That spotted cat of yours is real smart," people tell me, the newsboy or a neighbor who has recently observed Calico's rambles. "Why, do you know she always studies the traffic pattern before crossing a street, looks both ways, and never takes a chance?" She perfects her latent hunting skills and, disregarding the constraint that exists between us, comes often to the back door to show me what her swift paw and unerring eyes have won. As if performing a ritual she lays her latest prize at my feet: a mouse, a lizard, a sparrow. Carol tells me that Calico will sometimes capture a lizard, remove its tail, wrap the wriggling member in a leaf, and offer it to her, carrying the gift package in her mouth. She has even been seen washing her prizes, the lizards and small mice, dipping them gently in a puddle or fish pond and laying them out on leaves like so much wet laundry.

In spite of the rituals and the cleverness, Calico and I are still estranged. I am not drawn to her mysterious ways; and five cats are simply too many cats to care for. Paul agrees. Six days of vacation spent in a rented cottage at Laguna Beach, two bedrooms divided among five family members and five cats, are hectic enough to compel me toward action. I discuss the pet problem with a Mrs. Halleck, a cat-lover on the east side of town who makes a career out of finding placements for unwanted animals. She agrees to be an intermediary, Calico's friend and sponsor. For Calico must go, I am certain of this. Some submerged dislike of her stealthiness, her failure to be the companionable fireside cat of my imagination, surfaces in my mind. One morning I simply pick the tortoise-shell up from the back yard planter where she is sunning herself and begin driving across town. "Mrs. Halleck will find you a fine home," I tell her cajolingly. "You will always be provided for."

But the cat's wary eyes are on the half-opened car window and before I reach my destination she springs, struggles through the aperture and vanishes in the midst of a snarl of traffic. Astonished, I see her storming a distant curb, leaping upon a neighborhood of trim green and white frame houses, fences and cultivated rows of rhubarb and strawberries.

Hurriedly I park the car near one of the neat frame houses. What have I done? I ask myself. Am I not deserting a pet, releasing a domestic animal into strange territory? Isn't this act called animal abandonment, illegal, a misdemeanor or worse? Stories of abandoned cats and dogs, kittens left in parks and alleys, puppies placed on gravel driveways, in mail boxes and garbage cans, besiege my mind. The hills behind our house are often used as a dumping ground for animals, ruthlessly pushed from a passing car and left to shift for themselves. No one has been more critical of this cruel practice than I. "Calico!" I call in desperation, "Come back, please!" I tell her of my good intentions, how I mean to guarantee a secure future for her. But can she hear me?

Chastened and more than a little worried, I begin to search the locality. It is obvious from the milk dishes set beside porches and the surreptitious mewing and stretching going on upon the walls that cat-lovers occupy most of these modest homes. I knock at doors, introduce myself, gaze into sympathetic faces and enunciate the faltering question: "Have you seen a tortoise-shell cat run through your yard this morning?"

No one has. But I receive encouragement and advice; the cat-lovers are disposed to join me in combing the shrubbery and shouting Calico's name; several of them promise to set out dishes of her favorite cat food as bait if I want them to. "How awful this must be for you!" they exclaim sympathetically. "Tortoise-shells are so rare, such shy, lovely creatures!" They do not ask why Calico was riding in the car in the first place. They assume she and I are the best of friends.

Calico does not show up anywhere. I must go back home at last and confess to the role I have played in the mother cat's disappearance. "How is she going to survive?" the children wail. "How could you do this thing to Calico?" Carol weeps outright. She is not to be consoled by anything I say.

Amy, Carol and Julie join the hunt which stretches out for weeks, a period during which I undergo strong disapproval and antagonism from my daughters. I am thoroughly contrite by now but no true reconciliation is achieved until the day Calico herself resolves our tensions by appearing unexpectedly on the back patio—a rather worn-out cat, wearing leaves and seed pods in her parti-colored hair, deplorably thin, her copper eyes as alert as ever. She materializes on almost the exact brick where I had kidnapped her four weeks earlier.

"Calico's back! She's home!" the words ring out. We examine her and surmise the long ordeal she has withstood. It is easy to picture her weaving through cars and trucks finding the route back to the hills, living off the land, catching crickets and mice, existing one way or another, until she reaches security. "Don't ever, ever kidnap Calico again!" I am sternly told. Relieved and penitent, I promise. I keep my word. My respect for Calico has increased enormously; an affection for her is stirring within me. Calico and I come to terms, we accept our future together.

When the soft gray cat named Fuzzy dies of an intestinal disorder, Calico becomes Carol's cat. Carol is unashamedly sentimental, a prodigious mourner. She mounts a picture of Fuzzy on her bulletin board, keeps a swatch of gray hair, a whisker and a dried fur ball in a silver-covered cardboard box. She is the daughter who takes the Doctor Doolittle books seriously and asks: "Is there a language for animals, can I learn it?" She tells me Calico is magical, a true Halloween cat, and I am easily persuaded, readily won over now to this enigmatic and subtle being that Carol loves so lavishly. I grow used to Carol's attachments to horses and dogs; her quick rapport with the llamas that nuzzle her hands at the zoo; her scrutiny of hummingbirds and their small nests hidden in the flame trees, her preoccupation with frogs and wild rabbits and turtles.

"Mother, I want to be a surgeon when I grow up, but first of all I would like to be a veterinarian," she says, and I find room in my mind for this wish, allow the fantasy to mingle with the other fantasies I am already elaborating about my children, visualizing them as world travellers, ballerinas, editors—and a veterinarian, too, why not? The child's dream is certain to burgeon and yield fruit in the future.

Carol's illness, when it comes, alters these fantasies, changes our lives. She spends less time at home, is often at the City of Hope instead or in the company of friends, on the move, talking to people, living out the days. Calico and I spend time together. We become compatible, I losing my resentment, she giving up her reserve and skittishness. She is transformed from an outdoor cat back to a house cat again. At night she no longer sleeps on an avocado branch, but on the arm of a chair.

One afternoon Carol is at home resting, trying to overcome the usual nausea that follows treatment. She is content at the moment to be surrounded by beloved possessions: cushions and books, crossword puzzles, the fish swimming in their glass tank, Blackie at her feet, Calico within sight, preening herself on the driveway just beyond the patio window. Someone has sprinkled the back yard and Calico undertakes an enormous jump from the wet concrete to the top of the pink brick wall, a leap she has always been able to perform with sure gracefulness. But she is older now and cannot hold to the wall. Without a sound she slips, falls back onto the concrete and is killed instantly.

Carol's grief is more than I can bear. We weep together for Calico, for ourselves, for Carol. I shovel dirt at the top of the hill, burying the Halloween cat beside the white duck, the parakeet, the gray-haired fuzzy cat who was once Calico's young kitten. Carol is unable to watch. She goes to her room and lies down.

Later I come to her and we put our arms around each other and cry again, softly, persistently, each holding a revelation in her heart, each under a nimbus of truth, knowing we shall lie among these hills, too, in the earth's dark soil, some day, some day.

Chapter 11

Julie's short vacation in Oceanside ends. When she and I go next to the City of Hope we are laden with gifts, chrysanthemums, perfume, fruit, a miniature chess set. Carol smiles at us apathetically. The nurses are applying hot soaks to both her wrists. "Everything I do any more is a problem," she says. She points to a puffy upper lip. "I just pulled a piece of skin off this morning and my lip started to swell. So I put ice on it and a little ointment."

She is afraid the swollen lip or the gray dots on her legs will prevent her from leaving the hospital on this last day of treatment. "Everything is a problem," she repeats. "Even the tiniest scratch might be dangerous." Her moodiness deepens. "Mother, on television today there was a medical program and a doctor said thousands of people die each year from leukemia. Mother, will it happen to me?"

I feel my stomach transform into a stone, the breath leaves my body. I block out the immediate reactions, the sudden onset of fear, every thought except the blazing affirmation of John Donne's *Death, thou shalt die!* "No, oh no, no," I say emphatically. Julie's shocked voice joins in; she is even able to summon a reassuring smile. Carol looks from Julie's face to mine.

"Let's go home now, can we?" she begs. Her mercurial spirits rise. She packs up quickly, sits beside me in the small red Fiat, gingerly cradling the last wrist to receive an injection.

At home she whistles for Blackie. "My doggie, where is my Blackie? Du, Du! I'm here, I'm home!" She crouches to floor level, holds Blackie, releases him, frolics, gives him a handkerchief to growl at.

"Why do you call Blackie 'Du'?" I ask curiously.

"For the same reason I call Mousey 'Da' sometimes," Carol replies illogically. "Because it fits."

The phone rings. A neighbor impulsively suggests I take my daughter to Texas "where they are doing some really remarkable things with leukemia." She is yet another believer in the "breakthrough of modern medicine" we are hearing so much about.

"Thank you," I say politely, my eyes following Carol and the romping dog. "We are doing the very best we can. She is receiving good care and we have much hope." I do not mention the other suggestions people are making, the rumors and cures, the doctor who treats leukemia through hypnotism, the one who prescribes tonics, the clinics in New York, Mexico, Israel. I hang up the phone very slowly as if it were the rarest of heirlooms. I must deal with the unspeakable thought.... *but Carol's treatment is not really working. It is not working.* God! I cry inwardly. Where is the miracle? Send us the miracle, please!

Carol falls asleep on the sofa. As if lost, I wander quietly from living room to kitchen to back hall, bedroom to bedroom, a stranger in unknown surroundings, someone who finds a folded calendar on a table and opens it to discover the date. I feel only vaguely involved in this act, disinterested, like a figure from prehistory, a neolithic wanderer aware of seasonal change but unmindful of the individual flickerings of day and night. Tomorrow will be July 1, the calendar says.

I walk into the back bedroom and stare at the full-length mirror, seeing a woman encompassed by blue walls, haloed by a ceiling of dull ivory. "What if you start working again?" I ask the image. "Will you be less heavy-hearted? Can you still teach, do you remember anything about grammar and literature?"

"Just stay where you are," the image says. "You can never leave her."

"But a job in the world," I say. "Any job, answering a telephone, filing. I might become a stronger and a better person."

"No," the image answers. "No job can ease you. Do not expect any ease."

I tie myself like a knot at the foot of the bed and pray. Does someone hear me? I turn to the diary again, which is beginning to lecture. *Above everything else,* the diary instructs, *you need a preoccupation. Swimming and poetry and reading Tolkien are not enough. Look around, look at yourself, at your other earlier selves.*

The bedroom bookcase contains vestiges of the person who once studied languages, Latin, Greek, German, French; the high-school girl, the graduate student, the writer of short stories. A faded copy of Caesar's *Gallic Wars* leans beside Vergil. *Godwin's Greek Grammar* catches my eye, bound in maroon and peeling, one of my father's books that I used when translating Xenophon. Can I still translate?

Yes, I can still translate easy Latin, but I cannot find any Greek texts to decipher, only *Godwin's Grammar,* with its lists of verbs and dense metrical rules. The three volumes of *The Lord of the Rings* beam at me from the top of the filing cabinet as I write THALA across a sheet of paper, truncating *thalassa,* the Greek word for sea.

In my own fantasy, I tell Tolkien, the one I am just starting to invent, THALA is the name of an island set in the middle of a dark blue ocean, uncharted and stormy. A sailboat is being buffeted up and down the coast. I create names for the people on board, combining syllables from different Greek words, producing such hybrids as Zathos, Methomai, Apheu and Kraina. In search of atmosphere and action I re-read the legends, Roman as well as Greek, and renew contact with Lucretius and Homer and Plutarch in their English translations.

With a shock of recognition I turn to Plutarch's story of

Solon and Thales, two old wise men discussing marriage and the family almost three millennia ago. The designing Thales tricks Solon into believing that a son of his has died, that the funeral cortege, made up of all Athens, is even now being dispelled. Solon's bitter weeping and despair are followed by Thales' complacent moral, the justification for the lie: "Your anguish, O Solon, see how the loss of even one child can unman you.... This is precisely the reason why I do not marry and have children."

Carol is standing at the entrance to my bedroom. "Hi, mom. What are you up to?" she asks.

"Old books, history and stuff," I say, waving my hand at Vergil and putting Plutarch back on the shelf.

"Am I interrupting?" She grins. "Don't let me bother you. But I'm getting a real craving for tacos and brownies, both together. Do we have any?"

"Unfortunately, no." I regard her thoughtfully. "Tell me something, does the enovid cause this, do you think? I mean, bring on the cravings?"

"I don't know." She comes into the room, her long hair still tangled from sleeping, her eyes heavy.

"Carol, do you need any Midol?" I ask. "Are you cramping, is the flow worse?"

But I have over-stepped a boundary. She does not want to discuss any loss of blood with me. The effect that leukemia is having on the menstrual cycle, the sapping of energies, whether serious or negligible, are matters left to my imagination. "Do you talk to your doctor about this?" I persist. She shakes her head up and down, positively, agreeable but mute.

"Okay, honey, let's make a grocery list." I sigh, tear another sheet of paper from the writing pad. "First, tacos, then brownies—"

"Scratch the tacos," she says. "I've changed my mind. Can I have a tostada instead, a huge one? And stuffed olives, a chocolate milk-shake, and could I get green corn tamales, too?"

"Ye...sss, all this is possible," I assure her. "But it might take half an hour and in the meantime you will just have to starve. There's nothing in the refrigerator. Everybody was gone and—"

"I know, I know," she says. She holds up a small piece of yellow piqué. "I'm cutting out a top to take to Mammoth," she tells me. "Because I AM going there with the Spiris, mom. No one can stop me. I don't care what my blood count is."

I drop my stub of blue pencil. "Of course, Carol," I say, listening to it roll and crunch under my shoes. I scoop up a new pencil and the whole pad of writing paper and am halfway out the door, hurrying now, hoping the green corn tamales are still in season.

"Don't forget the brownies," Carol calls after me.

Chapter 12

"When is daddy coming home?" Carol, wrapped in the soft green robe, looks at me anxiously.

"Well, it depends upon what happens in Italy," I say. "Mainly on the strikes. He might be gone for another week, but it could possibly be a few days longer than that."

"But then he won't be here the next time—" Carol is interrupted by the ringing door bell and retreats to her room where I hear her hastily pushing the closet hangers back and forth, trying to decide what to wear.

The white-haired man at the door is Mr. Small, a deacon from Plymouth Church who phoned recently and offered to drop off some tapes and a book. While he and I are talking Carol hurtles through the room, pulled by an excited Blackie who tangles his leash and trips in the entry way. She waves to us both, leaving a wake behind her, an unmistakable impression of pallor and bright-eyed intensity.

"Mary, you need a miracle," Mr. Small says huskily after Carol and Blackie disappear. He hands me the tapes and the book, explaining that their author, Agnes Sanford, is a person of rare spirituality and healing gifts. He is careful in his choice of words at first, then grows more eloquent. "Miracles do happen," he says. "Miracles of faith occur every day through the power of the Holy Spirit at work in the world."

"But how does anybody...find..." my voice dwindles.

"The spiritual atmosphere around Carol is important," Mr. Small states. "There is much you can do. You can become a channel through which the current of the Holy Spirit flows." As he talks, a tide of memories rolls across me, past days and attitudes, the hours once given to memorizing texts at Bible school, Sunday mornings and evenings spent before the pulpit, the silent listening assemblages, alternately bored and attentive. The imagery of my visitor's persuasions is the familiar New Testament symbolism—dove, lamb, mustard seed, the tongues of flame and, permeating all these, the arresting figure of the healer whose outstretched hands succor the lame and the blind and those hopelessly ill.

"Faith is assurance," Mr. Small says quietly. "'The substance of things hoped for, the evidence of things not seen'." Never has the biblical definition of faith sounded so comforting to me. I learn that a Monday evening prayer group meets at the Smalls' home. "We have been praying regularly for Carol," the white-haired deacon says. He invites me to attend the group, then returns to the subjects of Agnes Sanford, visualization, the focus of healing and, once more, faith. At the moment of leaving Mr. Small rests one hand lightly on mine and says, "There *is* an adversary, you know."

"Yes," I say and thank him. As the door swings shut, a formidable question materializes almost instantly. What will happen to my daughter if my faith is not strong enough? The question resounds like doom, I cannot shake it off, or its companion burdens of guilt and human inadequacy, but regardless of apprehension I make a pledge. "I will try," I tell the closed door. "From now on I mean to dedicate myself."

Tolkien, I suddenly recall, creates his own version of the adversary. "However, my particular enemy," I say aloud, impulsively addressing that cautious Teutonic scholar, "does not happen to be your Dark Lord, professor. Anyway, darkness can't be evil, you should know that. Evil doesn't have any color." In spite of such convictions, I choose the title Leukos for my own adversary, selecting the Greek word for whiteness. "Leukos, the cruel killer within the blood," I announce to an empty living room. "I've named him. And he is here now."

I read Agnes Sanford's book, listen to the tapes and try to learn more about prayer. At the same time a profound restlessness drives me outdoors repeatedly where I rake up leaves, cultivate and cut back shrubs. And so, I reflect, the past is being renewed in me, because I am both my parents now, in a sense—my father, with his occasions of mystical intensity and my mother, working the soil, allying herself with the green plants, talking to them affectionately, as if they were so many diminutive children.

The fourth of July arrives. I go swimming. More and more I find myself turning to women friends who appear to be fashioning a supple chain of supportiveness, a linkage made up of many individual names—Michele, Roz, Sue, Carol, Betty, Jo Anne, Barbara, Joyce. One evening Jo Anne drives me to Laguna Beach; we pace the shore together, watching the ocean and sky merge into a sheet of dark slate. When I return Carol greets me with a question. "Mother," she says, "somebody called up about WASA. Do you still belong to that group?"

"Well, yes and no," I say vaguely.

But this kind of ambiguity will not suffice for Betty Brooks who is the founder of Women Against Sexual Abuse, an organization that is setting up a telephone hot line and providing counseling for rape victims. Betty wants me to remain an active member. I tell her I cannot.

"My energies are going somewhere else, life is more circumscribed for me now," I say.

Betty doesn't completely understand. I try to explain. "I didn't choose this, you know. It was given to me."

"Everyone has personal choice," she insists.

"Ye....s. Up to a point," I say. "But sometimes there really are limits. And I'm not being a martyr, either, if that's what you're afraid of," I say hastily in answer to my friend's quizzical look. "Right now I'm doing a lot of heavy thinking about both my parents, because each one—well, a kind of limit was imposed on each of them—"

Betty shakes her head.

"I'm caught up in their feelings somehow," I say desperately, "but I don't know if I can make that clear to you. There was my father's blindness, you see; he had to work within its limits. He learned how to live a circumscribed life, he had to."

But it is more difficult to speak about my mother. "Manic-depressive illness," I remark at last, "taught her the meaning of limits also. I have these two examples before me—my own parents. And now I've reached the place in my present life where choice stops. And the circumscribed life begins. So, you see," I conclude, "there is really just nothing else I can do."

No matter what activity I engage in, my mind accelerates. Whether I swim or write or launder clothes, broom the pink buds that fall from the flame trees on the patio, cook or type, I direct mental energy to the specific goal of Carol's healing, focusing on imagery and prayer, guided always by the suggestions of Agnes Sanford and others with exceptional psychic gifts. These efforts of mine are difficult to analyze rationally or describe even within the pages of a daily journal. *I feel I must live the attempt, become the exertion itself,* I write, stumbling after words. *I am hoping to develop into a human channel for the compassionate healing energy of the universe. A way exists, through images.*

The religious forms which appear upon my inner landscape nearly always derive from the natural world. And somehow the biblical fig tree unites with the small bent shape of the living fig that grows half-way up the hill, the New Testament dove becomes the commonplace bluejay circling overhead, the Rose of Sharon changes into the white gardenia I break off from the bush and lay on my palm.

Although imagery and prayer absorb me, Carol seems unaware of my concentration. She is helping Steve construct an outdoor aviary and as she comes and goes through the summer afternoons I hear her laugh more and more frequently or sing to herself. My sensitivity develops to a point where visual or auditory impressions possess a stunning power; the sound of a radio blaring comes to me blatant as an insult, the twittering of sparrows magnifies, is converted into the violin section of an orchestra. Within this new awareness thought vibrates like shafts of light.

Carol and Julie and I are grouped in front of the television set, watching a movie while Carol sews. She kneels beside the cutting board on the floor and pins flimsy strips of pattern to a rectangle of orange material. I am deeply conscious of the bruises on her legs, the marks left by the butterfly needles and the unnaturally pale skin. In accordance with the visualization techniques of the mystics and healers I pin one clear image after another of the healthy Carol over the signs of illness. As she secures paper to cloth, so I lay the contours of health upon the signature of leukemia. Carol, water-skiing, her head thrown back, body tanned, each muscle tensed and balanced against the opposing motion of the waves. The flushed and excited Carol of last February, a member of the mini-homecoming court at her high school, standing with fifteen other young women on the basketball floor of the gym, dressed in pink and carrying a long-stemmed scarlet rose. Another image, Carol exultantly climbing the observation tower at Door County, Wisconsin, her cheeks ruddy as the sunset flooding the twilight sky. I affix these pictures of a sparkling Carol over the one I see before me cutting and trimming the orange cloth; and I pray intensely for the former images to return. I live in this prayer and within the vital healthy likenesses I hold of her.

She looks up at me. "Tomorrow's Monday," she says, "and I'm supposed to go back to the City of Hope. Why isn't daddy home yet?"

"Don't worry, he'll come. I'm certain he'll be back before your treatment starts," I say calmly while I watch the glowing Carol of last summer rise up on the water skiis, then climb the dizzy plank steps of the observation tower. The Carol of six months ago meets my gaze with undisguised pleasure as she walks toward me across the basketball court and waves, tracing an arc on the air, brandishing her single scarlet rose.

Chapter 13

The repetitions unwind like a drum roll. "The blood isn't doing the great things we'd hoped for...it's not normalizing...more transfusions needed, more platelets." When Dr. Graham repeats "the leukemia isn't going to go away" I stare at her voicelessly. My mind insists *yes, it will go away, the miracle I am praying for will happen.* The doctor politely waves me past the office door, her face bland and uncomprehending; she cannot possibly guess my thoughts.

Treatment begins after supper. Birdie starts the wrist-tapping and vein-hunting. "Carol," I say, "did I tell you that our next-door neighbors had their trash barrels stolen yesterday? Can you imagine?" I plunge extravagantly into this flimsy story and am rewarded by hearing a soft gasp and "really?" Carol breathes, shifting her eyes from her wrist to my face.

The young nurses' aide named Jill March seizes Carol's attention next and spins a tale about Missouri and her childhood tribulations there, largely at the hands of "the fat kid" who, she says, one September day "just shot at me for no reason at all with his beebee gun...and I wound up picking lead out of my arm for months." Carol's jaw drops. Looking pleased with herself, Birdie successfully inserts the butterfly needle and the daunomycin pours down the inverted bottle and the tubing into Carol's wrist. Carol braces as if for an electrical jolt and closes her eyes.

Although we are anticipating Paul's return from Europe at any moment, it is still a surprise when he strolls calmly into Carol's room at 8:30. "Well, hello, hello, everybody, I'm back from Italy," he announces and smiles directly at Carol. She returns the smile radiantly. He kisses her cheek lightly, avoiding the I.V. apparatus.

"Oh, daddy, I've been hearing some really strange stories tonight," she says. "Everybody's telling me far-out things. Do you know any you could tell me, too?"

He does, of course; he has a few anecdotes about the hotels in Milan and their unpredictable telephone service. The three of us linger around Carol's bed inventing small talk and trying to disregard the glaze that slowly settles over her eyes.

The next morning I tell Paul the results of the last blood count and summarize Dr. Graham's discouraging report. He cannot disguise his shock. We eat breakfast together enveloped in a cloak of sadness. But the day, each day, must be gotten through; and Paul leaves for the plant clearly anticipating the challenges of business while I devote myself to routines different from his, the new patterns I am trying to create.

Reading about miracles and healing, I steep myself in the language and emotional tones of expectancy; I pray hard, exhausting myself. "Don't strain so much!" I order my laboring will. "Pretend it's just like learning how to execute a new dive. Let the muscles relax, wait for the lift from the diving board. Relax, relax. Let prayer flow." And saying these words, I pray more tensely than before.

When the mockingbird begins to sing from the top branches of an orange tree I open my diary and write: *It is the summer of the gardenia's profuse flowers and the mockingbird's music and the terror of Leukos.* I pull out my tablet of yellow notepaper and work on THALA, heightening the rage of the storm that is battering the island's coast and astounding the four people in their sailboat. On the leeward side of the island a possible port opens up for them, distinct glimpses of a sandy beach surrounded by basalt cliffs. But the four persons I am shaping behave like soft clay; they change in every sentence, will not stabilize, and after a while I abandon them to the sea around Thala, their characters and interests still formless and only vaguely intimating the classical qualities I am striving for.

Soon it is time to leave again. I drive alone to the City of Hope; near the midpoint of my journey the sign indicating a certain freeway turn-off settles tenaciously across my vision. The individual letters, white upon green, that spell LIVE OAK seem freighted with potency, nor is this the first occasion that I have been aware of their suggestion and power. The two words enter my consciousness, drum and reverberate, until I am possessed by them. I pronounce their syllables LIVE OAK, LIVE, LIVE so that they take on reality, substance, meaning. Dwelling upon these sounds is a means of ensuring my daughter's life—or so I tell myself brooding deeply within the resonance of each letter.

I switch on the car radio, am borne at once into the strains of a symphony orchestra, music which cascades large rounded drops of sound like globules of dew forming on a leaf edge. I seize one note, hold onto this single pure pulsation for as long as I can, extending its richness, refusing to let its vibrations sink into the welter of the other tones. Nothing, nothing must end, I whisper, nothing must end.

At the hospital Carol exhibits extreme depression. "Mother! I'm so tired of being sick!" she cries. "I'll never get well. Can't you just take me home?" She cannot eat or get dressed or even make her hair behave properly.

When Julie arrives at Wing Five both daughters unite in accusing me of tedious absentmindedness. I never remember the directions to the grocery store in Duarte, I get lost, I leave the car keys at the cafeteria. "Oh, mother, that's so *lame* of you," they chorus.

Julie goes home soon, but I stay on throughout Paul's subsequent visit and the frustrations of chemotherapy. At no point in the day does Carol's morale seem to improve. If I pass the time in her room she ignores me. If I leave, I must encounter her indignant glance. Any comment I make is, somehow, entirely wrong. "Shall I bring the telephone in?" I ask. "Would you like to walk to the T.V. lounge?" Carol shakes her head at me, or shuts her eyes to express disbelief at my obtuseness.

Treatment is over at last. When I finally pull out onto the Duarte roads my own mood is as dark as the black gaps that lie between the shiny punctuation points of the street lights. The sky seems covered with cobwebs; the freeway constricts like a tunnel. I am agitated by impulse, seized, convulsed by irrational forces. Just twist the steering wheel a little to the right, some element within me urges, now, now, here where the bank is steep. Why go through more, why watch Carol suffer? The frenzy passes. I keep to the freeway and drive and drive following the uncompromising route ahead.

At the City of Hope the next morning I am Carol's only visitor. A sympathetic nurse, Cathy Robinson, tells me gravely, "Carol's friends are having to adjust their own philosophies to this illness, too. It could happen to them, you know," she says giving me a direct look, "and they must face the very fact of that." Fear is keeping some young people away, the nurse is saying, caution, also, of course, the wish to protect Carol from possible infections, but primarily, fear inhibits them.

I walk into my daughter's room to encounter her stern and disconsolate gaze. Depression is upon her still; she will not be comforted. Wanting to express love and reassurance, I strangle in words. "What can I bring you right now, honey?" I ask hopefully. "Would you like some playing cards or a magazine or what?"

"Nothing," she says morosely.

"Some avocados, maybe?" I persist. "Chocolate ice cream? What about that?"

"Mother, I said nothing, don't bring me a thing, please." She turns her face away from mine, stares at the T.V. set. It is useless, she has no more to say. Eventually I leave and drive home battling a sense of failure.

"What's the matter with my approach?" I ask Julie. "What is it I am doing wrong?"

Julie says bluntly, "Mom, it's because you act as if she were really sick."

Here is the answer: fear shows. I must develop and wear a mask with features that are never disarranged, eyes that stay pleasant and unclouded, no matter how severely I struggle with Leukos and the fear he breeds. I must gain control and hold it. Every single day.

Chapter 14

Time lengthens, an almost visible morass of minutes and hours. I alternate between housework and writing, prepare the kitchen for the new vinyl tile that is to be laid soon, take Blackie to the veterinarian for a rabies shot, argue with Paul. We are both tense. He criticizes my selection of a sleeping bag. When a light bulb blows out above the sink he insists that I change it. "That's your responsibility," he says.

I retaliate by bringing up the air conditioning issue again. "It's hot and stuffy in every room," I remonstrate, "but especially in the front bedrooms." We reach an impasse. I sense he is suffering just as I am. Neither of us can handle the mounting stress; in our desperation we are rending each other.

Often it seems to me as if the members of my family are pacing about and encircling one another, spellbound and directionless; in these circumlocutions I see myself functioning like a sort of lightning rod that absorbs the hostility ranging through a charged atmosphere. The vulnerability of my position attracts every minute electric particle. I would like to counteract this process somehow.

One afternoon the words of a familiar Psalm heard over the radio in the context of a cantata, "I will lift up mine eyes to the mountains," move me to climb the heights behind the house, to trudge over winding roads until I can actually see the San Gabriel mountain chain north of the valley. The literalism of my behavior is obvious to me, yet I cannot keep from pleading with the distant peaks: "Give me courage! Show me how to live!" Across the canyons Mount Baldy, brilliant with snow and crimson sunlight, glowers at me.

Again I go back to the City of Hope. Overnight the hospital has been deluged by new arrivals. Men and women crowd around the admissions area; the corridors are blocked. To accommodate the influx a few leukemia patients are being transferred into the adjacent heart care unit. I watch them wander down the hall pulling their I.V. stands with them. Someone tries on a wig in front of a glass door scowling at the reflection and openly lamenting the loss of hair through chemotherapy. More patients emerge. Wing Five is flowing like an Interchange; people surge back and forth across the halls to greet each other and tell their stories.

Carol meets a young boy from San Pedro who is suffering from a unique blood disease. He fingers the scars on his neck, solemnly describing the surgery that produced them. The disease is affecting many of his internal organs, he says. Carol gulps at this disclosure. She is sharing room 607 with a pleasant Mexican woman, a grandmother whose swollen spleen makes her look heavy even in bed. The grandmother is resigned to her illness in a way that the boy is not. "Ah, I need transfusions, I can tell," she says tapping her stomach lightly. "And they want to take out this spleen, but I don't know, it seems scary..."

On this same crowded day we learn that Dr. Graham is planning a trip to Jamaica. "My father is quite ill," she explains. "I shall have to leave immediately." She becomes very direct with Carol stating the unpalatable truth, "Leukemia cannot be cured. You always go on needing treatment." It is a confrontation that Carol later describes to me with great effort. Tears brim her eyes. "So you see, mother, I'll always have to have treatment. I'll always be like this. Oh, mother!" she cries accusingly, as if I have been deceiving her all along about the seriousness of her predicament. And do I deceive her, have I done that? I rack my memory. Perhaps she is aware of my preoccupation with healing. Possibly the intenseness of my effort creates an aura of confidence which is now being destroyed.

"Oh, mother," Carol cries again, "see, this is how it *really* is," and "Oh, mother!" she says for the third time and, before the indictment I sense in her voice, I bow my head, face hidden, and let the lightning bolt strike where it will.

Carol does not see my unhappiness. "I'm running a temperature, do you know that?" The words rush from her pell-mell. "And Dr. Graham says I've had it ever since the beginning of this treatment; I must have come in with some kind of infection. And there's a lot of pain in my stomach, too, only she calls it my abdomen, and it's growing worse—but I can't get her to tell me why. She just says 'Some pain is important. Other pain is not.' I don't know what she means, mom." Carol pulls my head toward her, appropriates an ear. "What if it's my spleen?" she whispers faintly so that the grandmother in the next bed won't overhear the question. "And then I'll need to have surgery, my spleen cut out." Her tongue trips in a slight stammer. She is struggling with terror.

"Dr. Graham would tell you," I say quickly. "Why, if you needed surgery the doctor would surely say so. But she's never even mentioned your spleen. So it's all right, dear, of course it is. Try not to get panicked."

Jill walks into the room carrying a milkshake. "For you, lady," she says. Carol forgets her spleen and launches into a lively dialogue. I take a few moments to appraise the situation. How much there is to learn about Carol's reactions and my own! I think of my efforts at psychic healing: progress is slow, my tendency is to identify too closely with my daughter. What I need is objectivity, a more detached attitude. Empathy is not a help, it will undo me. And so I kiss Carol, matter-of-factly smiling at her puzzled glance and refusing to interrupt the conversation with Jill. I scribble a short note, place it on the bedstand and stroll out the door.

On the last night of treatment Carol's mood lightens.

"Mom, I'm feeling better," she confides. "I know I don't have any more temperature and tomorrow I'll be leaving for Mammoth and the mountains. Doctor Graham says I can go and you promised and so does daddy." She chatters on, her face suffused with pink, features clear-cut as if they were etched on diamond. "Oh, I'm so excited," she says, "but I want to be with my family, too. So maybe I'll fly home from the mountains a few days early, I think that's what I'll plan on doing."

I am back in favor, her beloved mother again. She jokes with the nurses, describing how odd she feels when a vein collapses, "like a little tube that goes pfft! And somehow all my veins are too narrow or deep or crinkled or something. Well, this disease just wasn't meant for me!" she concludes. We load the Fiat and go home.

Carol has been packing sporadically for days. Suitcases and purses and sweaters clutter the yellow bedroom while her mementoes, evoking every person or past event that has illuminated her life, spill from dresser and desk to the carpet. I see paper flowers, ornate and delicate rings, a baseball cap, rubber bands, a coconut shell, the needlepoint mouse she is working on, and "just how much of this are you packing?" I ask.

"Mom, I can't take everything," she says reasonably. "But I love all my things and they're so important and I really can't decide."

I attempt to close a bulging suitcase, extract a large stuffed panda and try again. "I think you'd pack the dresser in here, too, if you could, I honestly do."

"Can I take Blackie along?" she asks, her eyes snapping. "Please, mom, can I? I'll carry him in a picnic basket. The Spiris won't mind."

"The Spiris will mind," I say. "I hope the cottage is a big one. Wait till they see all your stuff. Please take out that shell collection; and just forget about Blackie's travels for the time being."

She falls asleep contentedly, primed to get up at five the

next morning, but the alarm doesn't go off and she wakes at 5:35, shivering in the cool dark. "Mother, I'm so cold," she pleads. "Please bring me some apple. I'm afraid I'm going to throw up."

I bring apples to her, sliced. Paul and I place the suitcases on the front porch along with a blanket, extra sweaters and her small wicker basket. We bundle her off into the warmth of the car that is waiting to drive north to the mountains.

Afterwards I drink tea in the kitchen, dress, and leave the house knowing I intend to go to church for the first time in many months. I walk through semi-darkness which is laden with chilly air and the muffled chirping of birds, enter a large empty stone building, find a pew and sit in silence.

KEEPSAKE

The beige box at the top of Carol's closet inscribed *My Travels* contains mementoes which by a fillip of the imagination could be converted into one of those chants the old railway conductors used to intone as they swayed down the aisles moving through the passenger cars: Wisconsin, Indiana, New York City, Vermont, New Hampshire, Colorado, Utah and—pulling across the borders of California—Lake Arrowhead, Mammoth, Laguna, Lake Tahoe.

The box holds treasures, relics, moments. The cardboard bottom is lined with the Sky Cradle Certificate signed by the flight attendants and the crew that flew Carol from Chicago to Los Angeles in 1957 when she was eleven months old. The winged cherubs and clouds of this document are obscured by a jumble of postcards from her natal city, shiny views of half-opened drawbridges, horses prancing down Wisconsin Avenue, breweries, botanical gardens, theatres; and by playbills of performances she has seen in Milwaukee, tourist buttons and pins from Indiana and Illinois.

"Did you throw out the broken Snoopy pin I was saving from the Marott Hotel in Indianapolis?" she demands one spring morning, happening to find me on the way to the trash barrels, my arms burdened with waste-baskets.

"Well, I may have," I say. A tempestuous search of the closet and the waste-baskets reveals that the Snoopy pin is indeed gone and I am to blame.

"Why did you do that?" she asks. "It means so much to me."

"But it was broken," I say, exonerating myself. "Why keep a damaged pin?"

"It was broken for a purpose!" she wails, refusing to tell me what the purpose might be or why she remains inconsolable for several days.

A few small sugar hearts carrying messages like *Come Dear* or *Ask Her* rattle loosely through the box, as do a green firecracker, a bar of soap from the Meridian Lodge and a plastic container that preserves all of Carol's baby teeth. A lavender booklet, *The Junior Guitarist*, symbolizes a seven months' interval of tense guitar practice. From the treasure-trove of her grandmother in Indianapolis comes a purple velvet case holding a tiny tube of perfume. Above the vial Carol scribbles a warning: *Don't break—for my wedding.*

Some incongruous objects are lodged in the corners—withered leaves, a cat's flea collar, wisps of grass from Lake Tahoe spilling out of an unsealed yellow envelope. The grass belongs with the crumpled gum wrapper and a label from a soda bottle, all of which commemorate a special vacation when Carol and Debbie, their freshman year behind them, stayed up for hours during long August nights to linger over beach fires, meet other sleepless campers and smoke clandestine cigarettes.

New York city finds a place in the beige box and Vermont and New Hampshire, stops along the journey that carried Carol across the country back in the early years while she was still gap-toothed and fidgety, somewhat reluctant to give up the backgammon and checkers games of the local recreation program for travelling. She joined her sisters in their orange and green flowered paper dresses, clutching straw purses painted a shining gilt and flew to New England. She rode horseback with her cousin Connie and swam in a pond that was altogether different from the ocean or the Great Lakes, a richly verdant body of water fed from natural springs, shallow, resonant with frogs and insects. She took back with her a single red stone, postcards and a handful of winged maple seeds to add to her growing hoard of memories.

Photographs become part of the record, glimpses of Boulder, Colorado, a December celebration that brought all the cousins and aunts and uncles together. She adds a gold and silver University of Colorado pennant, snapshots of Uncle Fred and Aunt Marion. And letters, too. After she and cousin Connie spend a couple of weeks in the Rockies attending Trojan Camp, the beige box is infiltrated by letters from campers. "Come back, Carol, come back next summer," one of the writers urges. "I liked you better than Duff or Candy..."

In 1972 Carol purchases an Instamatic camera which she proudly carries with her to Wisconsin, having decided to create her own photographs during the time she spends there, two weeks of an August lively and diversified, unblemished by illness, the last one to be so. When Julie and I meet her at the Milwaukee airport, the new camera is dangling about her neck; she chatters excitedly while we drive up the coast of Lake Michigan in the yellow Datsun belonging to Bea and Phil who are more than a continent away in Japan. We are headed north toward the peninsula of Door County which projects like a hitch-hiker's thumb into the waters of Michigan. The enormous lake sparkles, overflowing with breakers that charge westward like rows of unruly horses, white manes rearing and clashing, the pent-up energies dissipated over and over again in thin lines of foam criss-crossing the shore. Watching the spectacle of the waves, our own spirits antic and soaring, we feel that the blue diamond lake glitters for us, in some way belongs to us, as do the small car, the city we drive through, the whole of the state of Wisconsin and Door county itself.

"Stop! I want to take a picture!" Carol sings out at the first sight of the peninsula's fields of wild flowers, acres of queen anne's lace, goldenrod and purple asters. She adjusts the camera, sweeps its range to include a stand of silver birches whose parchment bark is peeling in miniature scrolls. We stop often to capture the dark northern forests, the fishing boats and piers, crumbling stone fences, a horizon suffused with startling rose-red clouds.

I take one photograph of Carol and Julie in a grove of cherry trees sitting beneath low branches which, having completed the cycle of bloom and the bearing of scarlet fruit, now support a heavy green foliage. The lighting in this picture is not quite right. The two sisters look into the camera, their smiles hesitant, subdued. The composition overstates the paleness and shadow, a kind of disharmony, Carol's face indistinct and glowing with the pallor of a moonstone.

The collecting impulse is upon her once more. She finds her trophies at Fish Creek and Sister Bay: pine cones, duck feathers, rocks, a gold matchbox from a Swedish restaurant—fishbones and toothpick, the relics of a fish boil in Egg Harbor. Her pockets rip, she pins and makes repairs and goes on filling them up. Happily, kindled by a reckless expanding enthusiasm, she hikes, climbs, swims, water-skiis, rows, eats, collects.

The last two days the peninsula mists over with light rain. Carol and Julie and I walk into the village of Ephraim and sit on a porch where we can watch the sailboats in the bay roll and dip under a shivering gray curtain. It is raining even more steadily the following afternoon when we drive to Cave Point on the peninsula's eastern side. Parking the yellow Datsun, we pace through falling rain to the edge of steep limestone cliffs and stare awe-stricken at the architecture that is being hammered out by the waves beneath us, the hollows and ledges, caverns and promontories, a ragged stone border embellishing the coast. No one speaks; the waves do the talking here.

Carol and I step under the tall pointed pine trees onto a carpet of thick needles. The wind follows us, levelling gusts of cold mist at our heads. We move back again to the cliff's edge and lean out to hear the hissing rain droplets strike the surface of the lake. Our lungs inhale the cool air that is so reminiscent of sea air, yet laden with contrast also, lacking salt, more redolent of growing weeds and minerals and earth, a true composite of freshwater smells. The restless powers in the lake rise, steam, explode.

Carol, mesmerized and preoccupied, for once forgets to pick up any memento from her surroundings; not so much as a leaf or berry finds its way into her pocket. No visible reminder of this place, then, will exist. It will be one of those moments of life for which memory is the only keepsake.

Intent, head angled to one side, she listens to the waves at work beneath the lip of earth we stand upon. "Crash, crash," the waves insist. "Boom, boom, boom" the caves respond. Does she hear anything else? The notes of the wind multiply. The shore birds cry out shrilly before racing away from the masses of rising water. Autumn is riding the bronze glint of these waves, behind autumn lurks winter: blue to gray to green to brown, the lake is in transit, passing through another of its immemorial phases—color, density, sound, rhythms, shapes, all in the act of change during this interval, this pause, a hush upon the heart, the last remaining stretch of summer before the storms.

Chapter 15

The postcard from Mammoth reads: *Dearest family—I finally made it! It is so pretty up here there are about 10 lakes & all kinds of scenry. I'm having alot of fun & don't want to come home! Tell Blackie HI! I guess I miss you guys! Thanks again for everything   Lots of Love, Carol*
    The exuberance of these lines does nothing to relieve my uneasiness. As I think about the matter, the entire trip becomes a haphazard undertaking; it is not clear whether Dr. Graham ever really gave her consent to Carol's plans. I have confidence in the Spiris, yet Mammoth seems very far away and the mountains a source of innumerable dangers.
    In order to moderate these misgivings I wash down the kitchen walls, squeezing the sponge with zeal and scrubbing anxiously at grease spots. The hot still air instantly consumes the watery traces my sponge leaves behind. "She will be home soon," I reassure myself at intervals, but this is not so.
    "Mother, I'm going to stay through the weekend," Carol announces cheerfully over long distance. When I gasp she counters "But...Dr. Graham isn't back anyhow, so it's O.K...."
    "You have another substitute doctor, you know," I remind her, "and the name is Dr. Kellon, remember him?"
    "Yeah. Well, but daddy *DID* give me extra money," Carol says defensively. "I know it's supposed to be for the

plane ticket and all that, but you guys won't care if I spend it on something else, will you? I can come home when the Spiris do."

The return trip is accordingly put off. I explain this change in plans to Paul who is preoccupied with the details of organizing a convention at Long Beach. "We're sending a man to England to run the plant over there for a couple of years," he says. "It's really very important. But don't worry," he insists, "I'll be right here on Sunday night when Carol gets back."

The house empties. I am racked by a spasm of tears, then a storm. My friend Shirley invites me to her home and gives me some magazine articles about the importance of positive thinking. People phone to ask about Carol. I attend a prayer meeting where I recognize many faces, women and men linked with volunteer groups of the past, with nursery school or grade school or scouting. In their sympathetic presence I keep back the tears, shutting my eyes and praying whenever my turn falls due.

One evening during the long week I follow the suggestions made by several people independently, neighbors and churchmen, and drive past the boundary lines of Whittier to attend a Charismatic service which is being held in a church traditionally Episcopalian. The rector, Father Landis, is more than willing to talk about the Charismatic Movement. "The historic mission of the Church," he says, "includes both preaching and healing." He relates how in the process of time the medical profession took over the healing function. "But now the Church is once again regaining its early ancient power to heal..."

As he speaks it becomes apparent to me that many Charismatics feel they are special, set apart from conventional congregations. Truly non-political, they follow goals which, in my opinion, could be called mystic. They belong to no one denomination, can be either Catholic or Protestant, and are sprinkled like citron through the large loaf cake of the Church: small earnest groups of people assembling in the sparse halls of out-of-the-way parish buildings or private homes. "A lot of church-goers," the rector muses, "want to have nothing to do with us. They think we are irrational, too...umm, different."

Some Charismatics also refer to themselves as Pentecostals, though this is making use of a very old term. "The word *Pentecost*," the clergyman explains, taking great pains with me, "refers to the day also known as Whitsunday or White Sunday and it commemorates the mystical descent of the Holy Spirit upon the Christians assembled in Jerusalem at the time of a traditional harvest festival." The event described in the book of Acts was said to be accompanied by supernatural signs: a great rushing wind, visible tufts of fire shaped like tongues or small plumes that settled upon the Disciples' foreheads, and the simultaneous gift of ecstatic speech. "You see," the rector goes on, "the Christians discovered they could instantly speak in the dialects of all the people who were present that day in Jerusalem...which means languages used in Persia, the many districts of Asia Minor, the Mediterranean islands, Alexandria and Rome. Which would normally be unthinkable, of course, indeed a miracle." Very soon after this spectacular occurrence the leading Disciples evidenced a miraculous ability to heal the sick, the lame and the blind.

Centuries of church history passed, wars, and the erosion of powers. "But today, here and now, within this century," he says emphatically, "under the impetus of the Holy Spirit, miracles of healing are occurring and the gifts of the Spirit are again revealing themselves. Glossolalia or speaking in tongues is just one of them."

In the soft light of the church chancel all things seem possible. Space takes on a miraculous texture. The laying on of hands, the priest's murmured blessing, the cross, the cup and the altar, breathe a promise of health and well being now, in this existence, and hope in a life to come.

Father Landis includes Carol's name among those pronounced during the ritual prayers for healing. After a very long pause I hear a remarkable singsong coming from the lips of the men and women who surround me, either kneeling or sitting in the pews. The strange tones quiver at first, then weave and climb together, separate into high clear strands and re-combine. "We are singing in tongues," someone whispers. A pleasurable shock jars me as I encounter this form of glossolalia for the first time, a spontaneous music which makes no use of words.

Minutes later at the altar rail the woman next to me utters a long moan followed by outcries so piercing I am sure the rector will intervene or reprove her. Nothing of the sort occurs. The pastor only beams in her direction and nods his head while the congregation takes no notice whatsoever.

Is a church service actually being conducted? I cannot tell. When the meeting ends people embrace and stand talking for long minutes. They ask how so-and-so is faring, what blessing has come your way? Carol's name is on their lips. Men and women smile, look in my eyes and promise: "We will pray for your daughter's healing. We love her."

And so I return again and again to these gatherings, to an attitude and an atmosphere that sustain hope and promote courage, my perceptions dazzled by the exotic syllables of those "speaking in tongues," a speech many would consider nonsense; and charmed by the singing voices that penetrate beyond the rational sphere into patterns of the unconscious, creating a beguiling mysterious music.

It is hard for me to break down the reserve of years but in time, I do. "It is *her life, her life,*" I think desperately, "and if this is the way, the course I should follow, I will follow it." At night I visit the small parish church and sit before the altar, knowing sadly I would seek out any power, pied piper, willow-the-wisp, any angel, fallen or risen, for Carol's sake. The meetings become my nourishment. I cannot stay away; and, eventually, almost without being aware, I, too, start to sing in tongues.

Carol comes home at last, clear-eyed and happy, her skin almost tawny. "Mom, do you know what?" she asks excitedly.

"There's a fissure, a F-I-S-S-U-R I think it is, running through the valley in Mammoth and it's filled with snow the entire time, everyone says. The Indians used to refrigerate food there. Isn't that neat?" She shows me color photos of mountains and lakes, huge rock piles and thick vegetation. "We caught 150 trout," she claims. "All of us did together, that is."

"Really," I murmur, not so much interested in the catch as I am in observing her. She parries my questions, reluctantly admits that her temperature rose once or twice; a lesion formed on one hip and burst. "I just used pressure and merthiolate and bandaids," she says, "and it's O.K. now, see for yourself." The skin is only faintly empurpled and does, indeed, seem healed.

"And that is the only thing that matters—healing," I tell Paul and Carol both, kissing them goodbye, having glanced at the photographs once again and sorted the laundry. I leave for church, intending to give thanks and lose myself in the strange wordless singing of the Charismatics.

In spite of positive thought or glossolalia, I am unprepared for the medical report that Dr. Kellon gives me the next day. "I said her blood count is *UP*, Mrs. Trautmann," he repeats, touching his ruff of beard which is tinged with the barest suggestion of gray. "She is making platelets and white cells on her own!" He is uncommonly tall, good-humored, with a ready smile, the single black member of the hematology team.

I stare unbelievingly at his approving face.

"And there's no sign of infection," he continues. "Even though treatment's been started, her blood count is already up!"

Over the phone I stammer a bit, first to Paul, then to Father Landis. "She's making white cells!" I exclaim. "And platelets, at last! Her own!" My excitement spreads to others; a glow of goodwill seems to bathe the hills and roadways, the very telephone wires, of the community I live in.

Unfortunately Carol herself is not in the least elated. Nausea and melancholy again distance her from us. She mutely accepts the bouquet of pink buds that Julie and I bring and bows her head while I fasten a small silver cross and chain around her throat. "Thank you very much," she says formally.

Paul would like to take Carol on a boat trip as soon as possible. It is his way of celebrating. He can find no reason for delay. "Not just yet," I plead. "Besides, where are we going exactly? Catalina or Point Vincente?" We fall into mild argument. "Catalina is too hard a trip just now," I say. "Sleeping on the deck all night would be too much." Paul disagrees. "She loves Catalina," he insists. Somehow the debate is diverted to the silk oak tree in front of the house which, he claims, is causing damage to the sewer pipes. "We ought to take that tree out," he says. I protest. "It's a dirty tree," he states, "and it sheds constantly. I'm surprised you admire it..."

The silk oak tree remains an unresolved issue, as does the boat trip. We cannot decide when to leave or exactly where to go.

Chapter 16

Released from the hospital again, Carol plunges into a spate of telephoning. A new school semester is to begin in September and she is beset by the need for making plans. In between calls she remarks casually that no blood transfusions of any kind were administered during this latest stay at the City of Hope. "No, none," she states firmly under my probing and she does not know why and she doesn't really care and would I please go away while she calls up all the senior song leaders? They have a lot to do.

"A lot of what to do?" I ask.

"You've forgotten we were elected senior song leaders? Debbie and me?" Carol asks incredulously. "How could you do that? It's very important and means a lot of work and responsibility. I have to get together with Debbie and Sandy and Janice and the others without any more of these stupid delays."

She's right, naturally I have forgotten entirely about the high school elections held last May when Carol first became ill. The politics of campaigning, the slogans, enthusiasm and suspense have departed my mind as if they never existed; even more remote is the memory of Carol's earlier attempts to win election during her freshman year. "We only lost by two votes that time," she reminds me. "Think of it. Just two votes. Me and Debbie, I mean. Debbie wanted a re-count, but we didn't, we waited until this year to run again."

"Debbie and I," I say automatically, but Carol is not heeding grammar. "We've got so much to do, honest, it's awful," she says, obviously enjoying the prospect of learning dance steps and songs, designing red and white costumes and making pom-poms.

"Then there's Hi Jinx," she rushes on. "When Club finally gets going on their skit and starts to practice, well, I'm intending to be in *THAT*, too. My friends are counting on me." She sends me a scalding glance, meant to convince me of her absolute commitment.

I realize how useless it is to ask her to slow down or suggest taking easier courses in school. My basic impulse, to keep her within a hermetically sealed bubble protected from any source of infection, has nothing whatsoever to do with Carol's human reality.

Furthermore, she has received another invitation to travel. The Spiris plan on renting a beach cottage at San Clemente near the end of the summer and, "They've got room for me, mom, they do," she insists, having already accepted their offer, determined that no hospital or parent will deter her. None does. "Well, O.K., Carol," Paul comments, "but I'm taking off for San Pedro to get the boat shaped up for you. So save some time for your old dad and the rest of us."

Father Landis is surprised to find me occupying the pews twice in one Sunday. It is actually the third service of the day for me, but I do not admit this fact, masking my panic and need, submerging the driving terror that impels me; instead I attempt to hold a brief theological debate with him. "There will always be differences among the churches," he says. "People just cannot agree on either matters of doctrine or ritual. So the churches themselves are always going to wear different labels. In spite of that fact, though, the Charismatic Movement is reducing our disagreements and uniting us all."

As for the misogyny of Saint Paul and the strictures against women matter-of-factly laid down within the New

Testament, the rector tranquilly refers me to "the historical circumstances and the customs of those days." Theological argument, social bias, even injustice seem inconsequential to me; the one thing that matters is healing.

"All healing comes from God," I say pointblank to Julie when I return home from the Charismatic services. To her the statement appears as a complete non sequitur. "Mother, you sound like a preacher," she says.

"But I thought you were glad to see me attend church," I reply.

"I just think somebody SHOULD," Julie answers. "Only please don't preach."

"But all healing *does* come from God," I insist to Julie's retreating back.

I am starting to publish again, after years of hurried and clandestine writing, the short stories, poems and dialogues kept tucked away in manila folders or between the pages of old magazines, the long periods of inertia and self-doubt. Some of the newly formed feminist journals are encouraging me. My poems are being accepted. In the quiet of the blue bedroom I compose laborious letters to editors, my fingers stiff and unpracticed, my eyes drifting from paper to typewriter to the tattered lining of the drapes that daily endure the sun's corrosive heat.

Carol enters the room softly. She has just washed her hair which streams down the back of her neck and drips through the pastel green of her robe. The towel which has been wound about her head in a loose turban hangs damply from one hand. I mean to greet her, but my daughter's dark eyes are fixed on the churning sea of leaves that toss outside the narrow window facing north where, through half-opened draperies, avocado boughs can be seen dipping, assailing the hillside; branches of the orange tree, pomegranate and sweet gum, too, near the ribboned and spatulate shapes of oleander and ginger lily. The words in my mouth fragment and dissolve.

Like acrobats or dancers rehearsing, I move away from

the typewriter and drop to the edge of the bed while she pauses, swivels and sinks diagonally across my lap. Her face is hidden except for a suggestion of cheek-bone and eyebrow. My fingers stroke her shoulders, the wet robe, a few strands of the hair that hangs heavily weighted by water and colored a deep amber.

She raises her head. Her arms tighten around my waist. We are both speechless, although bound within a palpable affection, two naiads or nymphs clinging together during a moment of emergence above the surface of a thundering river. Our gaze combines and sweeps the distance as if both of us were seeking some benison from this impermanent interlude of light and air. A current swirls, a whirlpool tugs. The river transforms to the wine-dark Aegean; the gustiness that sighs along the horizon is threaded with hesitant syllables not quite understood. Words break from my mouth at last, endearments barely whispered. "Oh beloved," I breathe. "My sweet child ...beloved."

Carol does not stir or answer. We remain tranced, drifting upon an ancient and consecrated sea. The gusty wind is more audible now, the hesitant syllables lengthen and become recognizable sounds. I think I understand them: Amphitrite, Creusa, Panope—the nymphs call out their names, including us in their gentle summons.

The waters plunge and fade and disappear within the blue carpeting on the bedroom floor. Carol rises wordlessly and leaves.

I am surprised when the following day occasions a number of letters and long distance phone calls. I had thought to ignore my July birthday, but Paul's mother telephones early in the morning from Beloit, Wisconsin. "I'm still expecting a visit from you this summer" she says to my alarm, in the voice that only now and then quavers enough to betray the fact of her eighty-eight years. Grandma, as we universally style her, knows nothing at all about Carol's illness, and, "She must *not be told*," Paul says shortly, the ever-present concern for his mother evident in the sudden wrinkles that groove his forehead. I comprehend his feelings, but the perplexing questions keep right on coming. How long can we hope to mystify this frail but very astute woman? Who is to be protected from knowledge, who not?

The same issue perturbs me when Amy calls from Milwaukee. Believing that no one has yet mentioned the word *leukemia* to her, I talk distractedly about pernicious anemia and the frequent need for blood transfusions.

"What can I do?" Amy asks. "Can I come home and see her?" I put her off, deliberately evasive, and eventually find, after considerable fencing, that I have promised to make a trip to Milwaukee at some indefinite future date.

The women's group I belong to convenes at my home and one friend, whose name happens to be Carol, gives me a recorder as a birthday present. "Sure, you can learn to play it," this Carol insists, running her fingers lightly up and down the instrument's polished shaft. "It might take a while, but you can do it."

Doubtfully I try to imitate her deft fingering. She has written down a series of musical notations which I puzzle over like cuneiform. Nor can I handle the evening's discussions with any more certainty. The topics—hitch-hiking, crisis center, rape—hover at the edge of my awareness, words whose meaning I am unable to absorb. I sense that I am brittle like glass and must protect myself from breakage, but who understands this?

"I'm really happy that you're getting on top of your own situation," Barbara says to me warmly and other voices concur. A wave of affection passes through me and then retreats; I am left stranded on a cliff like an abandoned pebble. The gorge below opens. My friends watch anxiously from the other side of an expanding gulf as the ground tilts and shivers. There is no way for me to steady the landscape, to stop the process of dislocation that is separating me from my friends. It is impossible to speak about the search I am engaged in, the terrible urgent need for healing that must take precedence over every other interest. Disconcerted, a little ambivalent and conscious of my inner fragility, I am just barely able to smile and thank my friends for their good will.

As the current end-of-the-summer plans unfold, both daughters approach me. Julie is going to attend a camp at Oceanside; Carol will leave soon for San Clemente. "Can I have the small blue suitcase?" they ask in unison. They each covet the new down-filled sleeping bag, too.

I hesitate. Angrily, Julie takes me aside. "Mother, just because Carol is sick now, you're giving her everything she wants and spoiling her rotten," she states.

"You don't mean that," I say.

"Oh, yes I do," Julie answers, brick-red and resentful.

"Well, let's draw straws," I say, resorting to an old unfailing method which neither daughter challenges. Someone finds a broom. Straws are pulled out and matched three times in quick succession before Julie accepts the sleeping bag and Carol begins to pack the small blue suitcase.

Chapter 17

"I am amazed that she can look so good." Dr. Graham, who has returned from her trip, studies Carol for a long moment. "Her hemoglobin is so very low. I'm surprised that she can even stand." Carol, pale beneath the suntan acquired during her San Clemente vacation, looks past the doctor toward the hospital orderly who is pushing a wheel chair around the corner—the one she has just been occupying, under duress, rebelliously.

"At any rate, better things are happening in other parts of the blood," the doctor says slowly with an intangible change of attitude. The crisp voice deepens. "We're going to give you some transfusions now, Carol, and then do another bone marrow. After that, we'll decide whether or not to continue this present treatment."

My daughter's gaze shifts to the doctor's face but she remains mute.

"You remember what I said when you first came here in May? That we might give you the same sort of treatment we use with children? Well, we still might. Though you certainly don't look like a child, Carol."

Ushered into her Wing Five bedroom for the transfusions, Carol says abruptly, "I have a feeling I might be in here for a long time." Her apparent stoicism changes to mournfulness. "A different kind of treatment? Does that mean I might not be able to go back to school?" She stares at me, her alarm full-blown.

"Trust your doctor, honey. Don't give in to worry, just believe in Dr. Graham." I can find nothing else to say and begin tugging at the curtains.

Carol has no appetite whatsoever. The diminished blood supply in her body causes a wave of giddiness to surge over her, through which I see her floundering; and the veins in her arms now seem further reduced in their dimensions so that none of the nurses is able to begin the first transfusion. Finally Dr. Graham is summoned; with a cautious economy of word and motion she at last finds the right place to insert the needle.

Paul telephones. "Your father's hung up in San Pedro," I tell Carol. "He can't make it through the traffic and will just have to visit you later on...but he sends lots of love." Carol receives the news with a slow nod and glowers at the dripping plastic bag above her head. "I've got to have three more of these darned things," she says grimly.

I hurry home and call my friends in Westwood, Hollywood, Whittier and Milwaukee. "You see," I tell each person, "if the bone marrow shows that this kind of treatment isn't working they're going to stop it and switch to something else, because no one really knows what will work or, in fact, if anything at all...can help." My sister in Milwaukee listens as do Roz and Michele and Barbara; they try to sound reassuring.

But assurance does not exist. I am promised nothing. In the room that is almost a blue eggshell I sink into my own mind and summon the well Carol; visualize her as completely unscathed by illness, a happy young woman who dangles a curl of red yarn under her cat's nose or pulls a pink camellia from the bush beneath her window.

I concentrate fiercely. In some region where thought still clings, a wish lingers: to meditate upon the Holy Spirit which I intuitively feel is an aspect of the sacred that contains nothing autocratic or judgmental, is no remote power needing to be placated, but something or someone generous and approachable. I do not know how to reach the sacred. I simply wait, holding to the image of Carol healed; entering a spacious country of the mind where dark and light alternate and clouds become rivers and rivers flickering stars.

With closed eyes and all thought suspended now, inwardly distanced beyond thought, I watch Carol's image recede. A current flecked with lights pursues its spiralling course, touches me, flows on. From its depths, sheer motion without form, then waves, ripples of quicksilver, the living silver from which form springs: a feather, a wing, a deer's eyes, the fingers of a woman. Shape-changer she is, features and outline at one time wind-blown or rugged; at another, statuesque and marbled, then veiled and secretive. She will not congeal or fixate. Her robes flow and change; even her hands are quicksilver movement.

She says nothing, tells me nothing, but brings the warmth of her presence. At the core of her fluidity rests a calm that enters my being and comforts me.

The next day a pleased Dr. Graham reports the good news: a truly satisfactory bone marrow test. "We are surprised and gratified, Mrs. Trautmann," she says. "We won't quit now, we won't change when we're winning!" I stammer an inadequate reply. Dr. Graham smiles and for the first time suggests the possibility of remission.

Remission! Carol is as joyful as I am, though feeling somewhat fuzzy and confused after the transfusions. Paul is notified at once; I drive home singing, eager to share this happiness. Everyone responds with joy and gives thanks in accordance with his or her individual interpretation. Some praise modern medicine, others prayer, the healing power of God or Nature.

The daunomycin treatment begins immediately on an upbeat, almost cheerful note. Birdie holds the green butterfly needle as if it were an arrow and remarks casually, "This vein over here looks all right, Carol," and launches the arrow at once. Carol doesn't wince and the vein *is* all right. She clenches my hand. Puncture marks on the right wrist left by earlier unsuccessful attempts are visible, but bruises are fading and small sores vanishing. At last, I think dizzily, her body is able to renew itself, at last, healing.

Paul and I talk about the boat trip, now a certainty, and settle on Catalina for a destination. "Steve is invited, too, by the way," I say. Carol would like to include the entire Spiri family but ruefully admits the limitations of deck space. She clashes theatrically with Julie over the fate of Blackie and the aquarium during her absence. "Who's going to take care of my angel fish? And the neon tetras? See, you're not even thinking of them!"

This sudden somber mood continues once Carol and I are on the freeway. My driving is making her nervous again, she says. "You have such an *unconscious* style of driving," she expostulates. "I can't believe it, mom, don't you see you need to move over into the next lane?" At home we go to our separate rooms, both edgy and close to tears.

She knocks on my door. "Daddy's still at the boat, isn't he?"

"Yes." I feel a brief twinge of envy. "He's fixing it up, getting it ready for the trip."

"This family sure has a lot of temperament," Carol says suddenly, and the tight knot of emotion inside me, the snarl of resentment, vulnerability and self pity, falls apart.

"Oh, Carol, please forgive me," I say putting my arms around her. She is still wearing the heparin lock in her wrist and at the sight of it my breath strangles. I hold her close.

Chapter 18

Cupping her hands, Carol calls to her father. "Hey, guess what, Steve just saw a flying fish go by. Look over there, starboard, I think it is." Paul stays inside the boat cabin, his hands gripping the wheel, while Julie and I pour out of the galley.

We examine the waves, ready to identify a pair of translucent wings skimming their surface. No such iridescence appears. "Umm," Paul comments through the open door. "I don't think anyone's sighted a flying fish in this channel for years. Maybe it was a gull."

Catalina Channel streams past shot through with spray and cloud, blankly devoid of sea life. Avalon Harbor is over-cast but crowded, sailboats and late summer visitors jockeying for space. A good many months have gone by since we last visited this island. As if observing some remembered rite we launch the dinghy, row, swim and shiver beneath towels and T-shirts. Speeding to the other side of Catalina we drop anchor in Little Cove and, once on land, begin exploring, looking for the legendary goats and buffalo, but finding only disgruntled quail in the underbrush and garnering a few shells and cactus apples from the sand dunes.

"We've all grown bigger," Julie concludes, struggling with the galley table. Various inserts and adjustments convert the structure into a rough sort of bed. "When are we going to get a boat that everybody can fit into?" Paul pretends not to hear. The trip is quickly over, a muted version of past visits when, sharing a fine exhilaration, we used to swim too long and too far out, imbibe too much sun and salt water, eat and laugh excessively. We are like swamp birds now, shielding a wounded member of the species; we huddle close, drowse against each other, protect ourselves from the pallor of the very one we guard.

Early the next day Paul tells me he is planning an immediate fishing trip with two boating friends. I feel the knotting of a tangled inner thread. "Six whole days!" I exclaim. "You're going to be gone that long? And just for chasing after marlin, which nobody even sees anymore, let alone catches? But how can you leave right now?"

Paul looks at me speechlessly.

"Don't you know how *hard* everything is?" I burst out. "How can you desert Carol? Am I to carry the stress by myself?"

He shrinks visibly, then rallies. "I carry it, too. Why are you trying to make me feel uncomfortable?" He accuses me of neuroses and hang-ups. "Just what am I supposed to do?"

"I don't know, I don't know, then go fishing!" I cry.

Paul leaves for the boat, I take out the manuscript of my fantasy and write a few pages to describe Thala, the windy island which under the inspiration of the moment becomes a peninsula. This island-peninsula, I decide, is all that remains in the Mediterranean following a nuclear holocaust. The world's continents are nudged together in a tortuous new alignment. "Everything will have to be re-named," I decide. "So let's begin." I glance at the Greek grammar book. Anagerno, a verb meaning to search, a good name for a river, the Danube's replacement. I invent more place names: Belos, a mountain, Melpo, Pelaxa, new deserts, deltas, tributaries. Thala, however, takes on the lineaments of Catalina as I write—tilted cliffs striped horizontally gray and white, rock or sand beaches, yellowing slopes studded with willows, a foreground of dark seething sea.

Dr. Graham is called out of the country again suddenly and Dr. Kellon once more replaces her. Evaluating Carol's blood tests, he says cheerily, "Hemoglobin is O.K. There are still a few blast cells around. We'll just keep on with the chemotherapy."

Returning home, Carol places strips of red and white dress material on the sewing machine. She glances up at me. "I'm going to miss daddy," she says. "I miss him already and he just left for the boat this morning. I bet he catches a whole lot of fish."

"Uh huh," I answer. A pulse-beat later I ask, "Carol, would you miss me if I went away for a week, too?"

She is startled. "Why do you say that? Mom, are you mad at daddy?"

"Not exactly," I say slowly. "I don't think that's exactly the right word." But there is no right word to describe the welter of emotions I feel. Studying Carol's sewing pattern as if it were the one item on earth that could hold my interest, I examine my feelings and recognize among them, jealousy. Well, then, jealousy or envy, consider it. I feel under-valued, slighted. I believe Carol has a preference for her father. I stand holding a scrap of the red and white fabric between my fingers and suffer anguish.

Are we rivals then, Paul and I, is some sort of current loose in the family, in the world, that pits us against each other? Is society telling Carol to value the male parent more than the female, and does she? I absorb the hurt of this thought without knowing why I experience such deep knife thrusts of pain.

We think back to our mothers...if we are women, Virginia Woolf once wrote. I do so now effortlessly, abandoning California and stepping onto a weathered concrete sidewalk in the Midwest. I bend down to pull a dandelion, touch the scarlet petals of the rambler roses that are weighting the white slats of the trellis fastened against a stucco wall. My mother's sun-burned hands plunge a trowel into the soil around the roots of the rose bushes. She lifts the thorny vines delicately. "But, mother," I am saying with impatience, "when will daddy be back home from the college?"

"Why?" she asks frowning.

"There's something I want to tell him," I say. I will not reveal to her what it is, I will not share my thoughts with her. All my will and emotion are fastened on the absent parent, the magnetic father whose return keeps me in suspense.

"But you wanted me to love you, isn't that the truth?" I say out loud. Carol hears and is bewildered. "What do you mean?" she asks.

"Oh, it's nothing, just a stray thought," I say, shaking my head with vexation. But this is not true, I am still communicating with the woman in the garden whose sun-burnt hands are breaking off the dried tufts of shattered roses. The yearning she feels sends a powerful flow down the branches of the scarlet ramblers that drenches and suffuses my own heart.

Haunted, goaded by the uncertainty that shadows Carol's face and by my own fear, I seek the Charismatics. On this particular Sunday evening, however, the program is different. I hear no ecstatic prayers or singing in tongues. A delegation of ministers and their wives from Australia occupy the front row pews in the dimly lit nave. Each minister addresses the assemblage in turn. I am made vaguely uneasy listening to the succession of cultured emphatic voices and watching the ministers' wives.

A critic yet lives within my brain, I discover, though my analytical faculty has been gentled and subdued for months. I know the critic is stirring. As the young Australians' voices rise and fall, in the very pause between two declamatory sentences, I feel my awareness bristle, take shape. It emerges, a spiny-shelled sea creature, a crustacean that goes by the name of murmex.

"You're angry," the murmex whispers. "You weren't expecting this. You don't think it's right for the men to talk continually while the women just sit in silence: not balanced, not democratic, not true to the whole picture of life, men and women *both* out there...but, in all honesty, hasn't this been going on for some time? What exactly have you noticed the women doing lately?"

"They sing, they play the piano, and they often speak in tongues," I answer. "They do that a lot."

"But nobody understands what they say," the murmex continues. "God may understand them but nobody else does."

"There are interpreters," I say indignantly. "People who interpret the strange speech. You know, interpreters."

"Who are they?" the spiny creature breathes.

"Why, uh...usually the older men of the congregation."

"Not usually," the murmex says, "*always.*"

My glance seeks out the cordon of silent ministers' wives. "Why aren't the wives ever allowed to speak?"

"It would certainly interrupt the program," the murmex demurs. "What do you expect them to say anyhow?"

"Women from Australia, a whole ocean away, their experience must be unusual and different from ours. Who knows what they could tell us?"

"But look at yourself," says the murmex. "Why do you ask the wives to say anything when you can't even stand up?"

I try to rise, defying this accusation, but the effort fails. My feet seem to be gripped by a steel trap. And the women who sit motionless in the front row are all wearing gags, I see that now. Fascinated, I follow the involuted windings of the habits and sophistries that bind their mouths. "I thought you'd notice, eventually," the murmex observes before its spines dissolve and the creature ribbons off into another portion of my brain.

In the morning I telephone a woman by the name of Lenore. She is a person who has the reputation of being devout and particularly gifted in her manner of praying in tongues. I ask her to be my telephone friend for a while.

"I need your help, Lenore," I say. "There is something I want to discuss with you."

"Yes?"

"About the Holy Spirit," I say. "We'll go into it later, shall we?" I hang up the phone.

Chapter 19

The grandmotherly woman in the bed next to Carol pulls her wrinkled top sheet until it stretches into a smooth white lawn under her chin. The blue eyes are considering a plastic envelope of blood that hangs from the I.V. stand between the two beds. "Oh, my dear," she remarks. "Do you really need to have one of these?"

Carol nods. She is watching the blood.

"Oh, my dear, you're much too young!"

Carol looks quizzical. Her roommate grows confidential. "I declare, you do encounter the strangest things in this place. Yesterday when I came in for my transfusion I saw a Hindu doctor give a shot of some sort to a Chinese infant. Imagine. And I met the sweetest little Philippino girl. Married, with a brand new tiny baby." Her voice drops to a whisper that can be heard down the hall. "She has *leukemia* of some kind and she's so frightened about it, what with the baby and everything. But I told her how they are doing such wonderful things with leukemia—"

Carol smiles. "Oh yes, that's certainly true," she says in an over-bright manner. The older woman has more to say, but subsides quickly when a rush of hospital personnel enters the room. Birdie, Jill, Dr. Kellon and an aide station themselves beside Carol's bed.

"Why, for heaven's sakes!" The disconcerted roommate

stares at me as a curtain is drawn around my daughter cutting off further communication. "Wha—what is she being treated for?"

I explain and the inquisitive face stiffens into the reaction we have all come to recognize—dismay, fright.

Paul drops by without warning having returned early from his fishing expedition, empty-handed and shrugging. "It was a dry run," he says, "but since the weather is still so good why don't we go for another junket in the boat?"

Before taking off again, though, we are told about the death of Paul's uncle in Wisconsin. Steve's grandmother also dies unexpectedly. These two deaths cast gloom over a dazzling sunlit September weekend and promote a subtle inertia that keeps us close to shore. We anchor off Point Vincente and stay there. No one even feels like swimming to the white rocky beach opposite the boat and exploring. Rather, we circle about the Chipsee with slow cautious strokes, wary of the sea.

When Carol comes home from school the next day she is brandishing a newly purchased pair of red shoes, the final item to complete her song leader's outfit. "Hey, you guys, *you guys!*" Her voice peals exultantly. "Guess what. Somebody is appointing me a T.A. in Homemaking. It must've been Mrs. Davis who recommended me. So what do you think of that? Mom, aren't you proud of your daughter?" She pirouettes on one foot.

"Well, of course, honey, congratulations," I say mildly.

"You don't sound very excited," Carol says. "I bet I know why. You never studied Homemaking, that's what it is. You were always into languages, English and stuff."

"Classics," I say. "Greek and—"

"Yeah. I know. Latin. But, mom, the high schools don't even offer Latin any more."

"Um. Yes. Well, now, I must have taken some courses in Homemaking." I ransack my memory. "My mother used to refer to the department of Domestic Science, that's what they called it in her day...."

Carol stares at me. A long pause materializes. "That reminds me," I say, uneasy beneath her exasperated gaze, "whatever happened your freshman year or whenever it was you tried to take that Industrial Arts class? You never would talk about it. You just suddenly dropped out."

She is diverted immediately. "Oh, gosh, it was awful. Do you really want to hear about it?"

"I always wondered what happened. Your father was pleased when you signed up for that course. He thinks you've got some of his mechanical ability; that's what he secretly believes. Parents do that, you know."

She looks stricken. "There were only two girls in the whole class, me and another girl."

"Another girl and I," I repeat automatically.

"And the other girl, I forget her name, dropped out the first week, but I stayed and tried to learn how to operate the power tools. And I did make some things, remember?"

I am able to recall a scoop and several cubes of layered plastic exhibited with a certain embarrassed pride.

"But the teacher hated me. He used to stare straight at me and say, 'O.K., you *fellas*, let's get started!' and then he'd glare. It was awful. He'd assign the lathes to the boys first and there wouldn't be any left over for me. I couldn't get my projects finished. I stuck it out for a month, maybe longer, and then dropped the course." She frowns. "He intended to flunk me."

"It would be different this year," I say. "Things are changing." That's absolutely true, I think to myself, but I also wryly acknowledge that no one today would deny Carol the Industrial Arts course or anything else she might hanker for.

"A lot of people seemed surprised to see me back in school. They—gawked at me." She gives herself a brisk shake as if warding off introspection and dashes to song practice.

The mounting tempos of Paul's business life carry him to the Midwest and New York state on the same weekend that Dr. Kellon pronounces Carol to be in genuine remission.

No doubt of it, the slides are normal. The doctor's good spirits reinforce the matter-of-fact premise I have never been able to embrace wholly: of course treatment works, this is how it's supposed to be, this is the way. No matter. She is in remission. I barely hear Dr. Kellon state that the drug daunomycin will be omitted from the next round of treatments. Carol smiles and tugs at my hand. We float home.

The hills reach out to me, insistent, loving. As I climb the brick steps behind the house I feel that I shall touch the sky. A pile of broken bricks at the top of the hillside lifts me closer to the heavens. I am ringed by a blue sphere and by green leaves, layer after layer, depth upon depth, and light, too, breaking from a core of soft darkness, a flickering candle-flame motion, heart of fire, the beaten gauze of it shivering forth to meet me, announcing the soon-to-be-seen fluent hands, molten gold blended with silver, and the look of joy that flames from a woman's image through change after change—pin-point, ripple, cluster, pivoting column. Who is she and why do I see her, recognize her and yet do not know her, are questions instantly consumed in the fierce constellation of joy that burns wherever I look—hill, tree and sky.

I go soon to share the good news with the Charismatics. They give thanks with fervor and conviction. Prayer is an invaluable adjunct to healing, they say, the waters of the Holy Spirit have renewed my daughter. I am urged to attend study groups which will explore the gifts of the Spirit further. Yet, as the evening unfolds, I understand that the hymns being sung and the prayers being spoken are not addressed to a Spirit but to a Lord, a King and Ruler. This language is not new to me: I know the redoubtable old hymns, have sung them many times over as a child. But tonight I hear the words differently, with perceptions called forth by the critic in my mind, the murmex, who appears whether I want it to or not, and points out the emblems of power in each succeeding phrase: crown and sceptre, warrior and battle, mighty throne.

And I am made uncomfortable by words. My distress

grows until at last I fall silent. The reality is that I cannot myself address a King or a Lord. I am unable to worship power under any form, however titled; it is an impossibility.

Afterwards, in desperation I telephone Lenore and we talk for a few minutes about glossalalia, though she does not use this term. She speaks, rather, of a "beautiful secret language."

"When you pray to the Holy Spirit," I ask her, "how do you picture it? What image comes to mind?"

Lenore is silent. "Did you say 'it'?" she asks cautiously.

"Well, yes, I did."

"Oh, my dear, that will never do. You must always refer to the Holy Spirit as He."

"Why?"

"Mary, the Holy Spirit is He. It's always been that way. My father, who was a very devout man, taught me that. You must always think of the Spirit as He." To Lenore the subject is closed.

The issue stays active with me, though. I reflect frequently upon the matter and finally work out a compromise for myself, invent special techniques to avoid using a personal pronoun altogether when referring to deity; or appeal to God directly through the second person, You. The Charismatics are unaware of my struggle with the pronouns, nor do they notice how sparing I become with the vocabulary of kingship and power.

Whenever I am alone such subterfuge disappears. Thought and feeling prepare me more and more often for the emergence of the flowing figure who seems to derive variously from solitude and darkness or from inner sources of light, stillness as well as motion, and whose presence brings a warm vitality spilling over into my life.

THE CHIPSEE

At sea water and sky engulf each other, merge in a blue silver continuum that arches like a great bowl overhead and creates a hollow echo chamber to catch and reflect sounds which come back from the blue dome magnified, distorted or heightened, even on a calm day when the wind idles. Always, aboard the Chipsee, I am aware of sound.

The boat is already ten years old when Paul acquires it. The two large engines concealed below the teakwood deck perpetuate a throbbing leonine vibration that acts as a continual background accompaniment. Conversations must be exaggerated, radio broadcasts turned up more loudly than on land. Verbal requests are shouted or pantomimed when the Chipsee puts out to sea, waves splashing noisily against her bow, birds shrieking from the air.

The boat lapses into silence only when it is anchored or moored. Neatly secured within a slip at San Pedro harbor, with white hull and aqua trim, the Chipsee seems out of place at first among her neighbors—a couple of blunt-nosed scowlike vessels and a dilapidated sailboat across the way inhabited by a recluse who keep a light burning deep within the cabin. We do not linger about the congested dock area any longer than necessary or on the gangway where the dense water gleams below the pilings flecked with oil and an occasional moribund fish or armored crab. We jump across barnacle-encrusted planks and coils of rope onto the Chipsee's deck grabbing hold of the gunnels. Already rocking to the relentless meter of the engines, we face tuna canneries and mast works that are also rocking while the boat backs out of its narrow slip.

As soon as the harbor breakwater is left behind Carol asks, "When can I drive the boat? Can I start now, please?"

Paul grins through a layer of suntan lotion. "You don't *drive* a boat, Carol," he says.

"You steer a boat," I tell her.

"You pilot a boat," Paul says.

"O.K., but when can I start?" Carol insists, standing next to her father on the flying bridge, which is the apex, the very pinnacle of command where the mariner meets the elements directly, whether sun, cold, wind or salt spray. Below, buttoned inside snug-fitting sliding cabin doors are the accommodations necessary to maintain life—cooking galley, collapsable table, the small V-bunks for sleep. The flying bridge transcends cabin and deck; with opaque windshield glinting in the sun and twin marlin poles swaying like antennae at either side, it flings a spacious window open upon the curved and turning globe of the world.

A grandiose view, not anything like the perspective seen through a porthole, I think as I climb the teakwood ladder to glance at the lambent horizon and put some distance between myself and the thrusting engines. "Reminds me of an orchestra somehow," I comment into the whistling air as the boat engages the open sea, engines full throttle, companioned by loud gulls and waves. Like timpani accents issue from the galley where cutlery is sliding among the drawers and the blue plastic cups are rattling and swinging against each other. Strident and clear across these sounds the ship's bell rings repeatedly.

Amy and Julie follow me up the ladder, their eyes fastened on the saffron and orange sunrise. At midchannel we pass schools of porpoises and flying fish skimming the watery surface. By the time we reach Avalon harbor we have each taken a turn at the wheel of the flying bridge, our hair streaming from our scalps, feeling the dawn mist give way to the sun. When Paul hovers nervously above Amy who is bearing down on a sailboat, she laughs at him. "Keep cool, dad," she says. Paul has put on his ancient navy executive officer's jacket; his grip clamps firmly over each new pilot's hands as we consecutively steer a wobbly course to the west.

At Avalon the duty changes. We must struggle through the maneuvers of mooring, leaning far over the boat's bow to catch the slender slippery wand attached to a buoy, scraping our knuckles, burning our feet on the deck which heats up and holds the heat. We inflate the yellow rubber dinghy as rapidly as possible and desert the warm silent boat for the Santa Catalina beaches. Once ashore we wave back to Paul, calling out "Hello—hello there" across the assemblage of sailboats and yachts lying within one concentric ring after another, the catamarans, the dinghies and paddle boards. Paul stands on the deck which has contracted to a tiny rectangle; concentrating, splicing a rope, he gestures toward us absent-mindedly.

Amy, Carol and Julie hike into Avalon. Eager to test the cool waters of the bay I dive from a pier just below the circular red-roofed casino. The waves close over my ears; at once I am catapulted into an underwater realm of dazzling clarity which glows like a flawless turquoise, deep blue-green. The sea swells and I rock with it, brushing the fluted edges of dark kelp that ribbons up from great depths. Moss-lined stones appear to be just within reach of my thrashing feet, but the impression is illusory, I cannot touch the boulders lying fathoms below any more than I can feel the skin of the large golden fish emerging from behind a grove of purple fans.

My churning feet are creating the only sound in this still opalescent world. Perhaps the fish are sensitive to the vibrations I am making because they swim directly beneath my body as if attached to my sea-shadow. In the transparent blue water I can glimpse the dark iris of the fish eye, the orange lacework of scales. Slowly the fish and I swim together inventing our own water ballet movements; we are inseparable until I gain the stern of the Chipsee. Then the fish scuttle off toward a moss bank winking like jewels.

"Did you see the fish?" I gasp as I stand dripping on the deck. "Bright gold ones. About eight inches long, bigger than any goldfish I've ever seen."

"Oh, yeah," Paul says. "Garibaldi fish. They're perch, salt-water perch."

"They're just beautiful," I say, "and they swam with me all the way from shore." Just like a bevy of escorts, I think to myself, or, no, more like guides.

The trio of daughters returns from Avalon and before long the noise of the Chipsee's engines ricochets from the sheer walls of the palisades on the island's windward side, alarms the seals clustered in the south and echoes again over the choppy waters of the channel.

The swaying vociferous Chipsee takes us many places during the next handful of years. Often we cruise Los Angeles harbor while Paul reduces the boat's speed and turns narrator, pointing out the designs of the ships in port, their countries of origin and probable cargoes. "Here's the fake Golden Gate bridge." Carol's flourishing arm indicates a distant span of green arches. We draw close to a burned-out tanker, a vast cargo ship flying Swedish flags. One by one we pilot the Chipsee past breakwaters and under bridges.

Sometimes the power boat carries us north a few miles to Point Vincente. Here we drop anchor and swim through weed and, like as not, stinging jellyfish, reaching a shell-strewn rocky beach in the shadow of the skeletal remains of a tall broken-down pier. Limping over the sharp stones we discover a sea cave, the still glistening pockets of briny water lined with starfish, anemones and purple urchins. We return whenever we can, though, to Catalina, the island where the Chipsee rolls and tugs pinned momentarily in place opposite bluffs and beaches, Emerald Bay, Goat Harbor, China Point or unnamed strips of sand where only gray terns call out a greeting and the surf rolls continually, offering shells and pebbles to the tideline.

One afternoon following a very rough channel crossing, a buffeting by rain and winds and the commingled uproar of fog horns and high waves, we anchor with relief in a secluded and unfamiliar cove. As the engines subside the complexion of the day gradually changes from raucous disorder to brooding calm. The sun reappears, the surface of the sea smoothes out. Amy, Carol and Julie cannot wait to row ashore in the dinghy while Paul, donning his skin-diver's wet suit and oxygen tanks, sinks underneath the Chipsee's hull to examine the propellers.

I lower myself into the water and swim a leisurely backstroke in front of the unknown cove but soon return to stand upon the deck and watch the sea grow copper-colored from the sun's rays. The storm has ended. I am alone. The binoculars I raise to my eyes can find no trace of another human being's presence; the lenses magnify stones and sand, the façade of a cliff misted over with cottonwood trees. The water horizon dips eerily, empty also, the dinghy vanished like a yellow speck absorbed in the green dye bath of the sea.

All at once I am stunned by the silences emanating from sea and sky and boat. Even the waves abate, they seem to stiffen into a plate of polished metal, their ripples soundless. No sounds issue from the Chipsee, either, which rides straight above its anchor chain, hushed, motors silent, without a breath of wind shaking the marlin poles or the ship's bell into audible life.

Panic invades me. "Where is everyone?" I whisper. "Why don't you say something?" I ask. "Make a noise! Say something!" My spoken syllables are swallowed up by the dense calm which deepens and deepens, as if part of the sea itself, that formless mysterious element whose rollicking vari-colored surface can gloss over chaos and loss of identity.

Stupified by the mocking quality of this soundlessness, challenged by the harsh glitter, I lean out from a gunnel, poised to dive and ready to search the wide strip of coppery ocean below. Before my feet can leave the edge I hear the splash of oars dipping in water and to my delight the dinghy rounds a spit of rock. At the same time Paul's masked head emerges. Seconds later voices ring out, laughter peals. Soon the engines start up. The unknown recedes, the familiar is regained with all its noisy cacophony and emphasis.

"Hey, mom," Carol cries, "see what I brought you." She places a long piece of seaweed in my hand, dark blue-green, its coils strung with tough tight air-filled sacs like large pearls. "Just listen to this." Carol's finger-nail punctures one of the sacs. Air rushes out explosively.

"Isn't nature great?" she asks. "See. These are little

built-in life preservers, just like the big orange ones daddy keeps in the locker up there." She waves toward the bridge. "Well, this plant's even better, it's got buoys stuck all over holding it up all the time so the plant won't ever sink too far or get lost or anything. The buoys will support it forever, no matter what." She pops two more of the sacs before winding the damp leaves around my wrist in a bracelet. I stare with astonishment at the tough green globules spaced within the algae. "You're giving me a life preserver?" I ask.

Carol nods. She is pleased with her trophy. "Not all the seaweed has these little buoys, but this kind does. Want me to make a wreath out of it?"

"Thanks, Carol," I say. "It's just fine the way it is. I like it: a genuine float from the sea."

The Chipsee's last harbor cruise is recorded on a tape that is made on Christmas Day, 1974. The tape begins with a burst of noise. The listener can distinguish the pounding engines, a contrapuntal stream of radio music, occasional singing. Against this background Carol and Paul can be heard conversing, their voices distinct at moments, then diffused, taken up into the depths of other sounds. Fragments of talk flash brightly, phrases and words about travel, skindiving, lost cargo, accidents at sea, driftwood, the Morse code. The tape drones on. Carol takes her turn at steering. "You missed that by about fifty feet," Paul's voice calls out. "Aim where the other boat is, Carol, right at the end of the blue warehouse." Carol pilots the boat, Paul instructs, the tape goes on and on while the music flows and the cabin door opens and slams shut, opens and closes.

The diverse sounds of this tape whenever I listen to them induce a dreamlike hypnotic effect. As soon as the engines begin throbbing I seem to stand on the flying bridge along with the other members of my family. The air mists, then grows balmy. It is no longer Christmas, it is summer. The Chipsee leaves the harbor and the breakwaters behind, draws close to the turquoise shelf of the familiar island. Through the clear ocean currents encircling the shores I can glimpse a convoy of golden garibaldi fish swimming in their full beauty and strength. They move delicately just ahead of me, pilots and guides, past pale threat and dark submerged ruins, and I see that the boat is being supported in its progress by more than the ocean current, it is lifted and carried forward by the twining arms, the pale green jeweled air sacs and stanchions of the buoyant and enduring kelp.

Chapter 20

The kitchen drawer rattles as Carol's fingers search its contents; the upper cupboard doors open and close shut.

"What are you looking for?" I ask.

"The little red book," Carol says solemnly. Her summertime pets, the two hermit crabs and the turtle, are packed tight in a cardboard box and surrounded by cotton. They are dead, I realize with a catch in my throat, and she is laying them out for burial.

"But what happened to them?" The terrarium, a glass cubicle lined with sand and cactus, sits bleakly on the counter top. "Didn't they get enough water?"

She shakes her head. "I don't know," she manages to answer. From a deep drawer near the sink her hand extracts a red doll-sized booklet with Bible verses printed inside, a prayer book for her pets, part of the ritual she is inventing.

I follow her outdoors. Debbie waits next to the fence, hands folded, patiently studying the grave that has already been dug in the adobe soil. Carol proceeds with her order of service, prays, scatters hibiscus flowers and reads from the booklet: "Oh, death where is thy sting? Oh, grave where is thy victory? Blessed are the pure in heart for they shall see God."

The day is blighted for her; she does not really regain her sparkle until the next afternoon when the results of the high school varsity club vote are made public. She will be one of the twenty-two contestants running for Homecoming Court. Astonished and delighted, she shouts: "Me and Debbie! They chose me and Debbie! And twenty other girls!"

The phone rings. "Well, it's a gradual process, I gather," I try to explain to my sister who calls long distance. "You and I don't understand this sort of thing at all; I mean, did we even *go* to Homecoming in high school? But out here it's a big event. The varsity club actually selects twenty-two girls from the student body and—well, all the boys in school vote about a week later and they elect seven to be on Homecoming Court." I draw a guarded breath. "And I don't know exactly how it's done, but from the final seven a queen is chosen and two princesses and the other girls—"

"Do you mean to tell me Carol is interested in this?"

"Well, but, honestly, they all are. What can anybody do? It's not like high school back in the Midwest twenty-five years ago!"

"But what's the appeal?" my sister demands.

"Oh, I guess it's just the excitement. The publicity, write-ups in the school paper and the photographs."

"It's competitive," Bea says flatly. "The only thing I can ever remember about Homecoming was that it took place two weeks before Halloween. And Halloween was better, it was a lot more fun."

"Yes, I know. But, you see, this year Carol's so involved. Senior Council and things. Activities are good for her. I mean supportive."

A pause. "Well, if she likes it. We're just awfully glad to hear she's in remission." Another pause. "Do you think this might be an appropriate time for you to come to Wisconsin?"

And so it is arranged that my trip to the Midwest will follow hard on the heels of Paul's recent visit there. I shall see Amy and Grandma and escape Homecoming.

Carol is disgusted with me but at the same time too rushed and preoccupied to make many objections. "I guess you're still not going to let Grandma know I'm sick," she says waiting in the out-patient clinic at the City of Hope. We are summoned into the office before I can respond.

Treatment is much simpler now. No daunomycin, no I.V. hanging overhead, only the narrow lance of the butterfly needle ushering the cytosine into her wrists. She still turns to me and grabs my hand just as before, and I stroke her gently.

Dr. Kellon wants to talk to Carol privately. While they are sequestered together, a large man, a truck driver and cancer patient, tells me his story. He does not thank God for his own remission; he thanks the City of Hope. "This place has kept me alive for three years," he says. "I sure hope they do as much for your daughter. See, now, she's been given a second chance."

A second chance. That's how the big man looks at it. But this is not enough, no half-way measure can suffice, not where Carol's life is concerned. Only healing, recovery, the gift of normality, to be like other well people. With dry mouth and closed eyes I sit on a bench and pray for Carol to be exactly as she was one year ago. Exactly. Holy Spirit, please heal her, I breathe.

A businessman in Whittier, someone I have never met, telephones to comment upon my daughter's "recovery, the miracle," he says. "I would just like for you to know we find her example an inspiration and we are grateful." Someone else calls to tell me that Tolkien has died. The news takes me off-balance, while I am in the midst of packing for Wisconsin.

The Tolkien Reader lies open on a shelf at my elbow. I have been reading some of the rollicking verses and *Leaf by Niggle*. Tears cloud my eyes. A beloved grandfatherly figure has walked out of my life—that is how I feel. I drop a pair of shoes on the lid of my suitcase and go through a ruthless bout of self-confrontation.

The murmex re-appears, rumbling with accusations and asking unfriendly questions. Why are you trying to write a fantasy, anyway? it demands. Your life, nothing but inconsistencies, a hodge-podge of experiences. What, after all, do a mere four years' study of classical languages amount to? And so long ago, besides. You don't want to admit how long. Tolkien based his fantasies on a lifetime of scholarship, undeviating, perfectly integrated. His writing, a pure unseamed robe. I suspect your fantasy, says the murmex, would turn out to be a crazy quilt.

To the diary I confide: *I wish I were a Charlotte or an Emily Bronte—and am not. I wish I could be a female Tolkien—and can not. I shall have to be who I am, myself, and do the best I can with her.* I compose one final paragraph in *Thala* suspending its action forever. The island vibrates with thunder, surf and wind, the clatter of a smashed boat battering the reefs. My survivors climb up from the beach and pull themselves through the low mountain passes. Another person has been added to the original cast of four characters, a kindly old man with the air of a don. Near-sighted, peering at the blue-tiered mountains, pipe in hand, he could be JRR Tolkien or just as easily my own father.

Chapter 21

I'm north again. The winds from Canada blow trumpet blasts across the great lake. The shrubbery in the park tosses as it is divested of a trembling burden of red-brown leaves. High on the city's bluffs I am enfolded by the colors of Indian summer, a clear heady scarlet, the golden pyres of oaks, maples stained the pure orange that stuns the eye. Below me where the lake wrinkles and crawls, more color outpours. Like yards of gleaming silk released from enormous rollers, the waves advance in azure and jade green swathes to pile and tangle along the breakwaters.

My oldest daughter walks with me through the blazing park and tells me how much she wants to come home. "I haven't seen Carol since this thing happened," she says somberly. "I know my grandma likes having me nearby and my aunt and uncle have been real nice, but I would like to see my sister." We pass clumps of red canna lilies and borders of pink and orange zinnias set in the park's bright green grass, and plan for the future: Amy to return, the five of us to be reunited during the Christmas holidays.

Immersed in the glossy panorama of a midwestern autumn, meeting old friends, holding diplomatic conversations with Paul's mother, I forget about Homecoming. Paul quickly reminds me. "Carol is a princess!" His normally controlled voice wobbles unsteadily across two thousand miles of prairie and mountain.

An even more excited voice interrupts. "Debbie got elected queen! And I'm her princess!"

"You missed Carol's big moment," Paul insists loudly and by now everyone is gathered about the telephone—Amy, my sister and brother-in-law. "It was just great, you and Amy should have been here!"

Though I am unable to get the sequence straight, the big moment, it appears, occurred when the queen and her two princesses were crowned with rhinestone tiaras, applauded and driven around the football field in an open convertible. I close my eyes and see Carol waving to the stands. I wonder if she was warm enough that evening or if she has developed an infection, is bluffing, and needs an antibiotic.

"Hi again, mom! So what do you think of your dear daughter now?"

"Congratulations. It's wonderful." The telephone is passed from hand to hand until the subject wears thin. "The excitement will soon die down," I say confidently to the others in the sunlit kitchen. The ensuing months prove how exactly wrong I am, and how inaccurate this facile prediction.

Homecoming lasts all year I discover to my amazement. Far from being concluded by a football game and band music, the event is prolonged through publicity and kept alive in meetings and assemblies until June graduation. There are constant reminders: pictures of Carol and the court in formal dress, in short skirts or slacks, striking a variety of poses, clowning, looking comic or serious and sedate. The phone rings more than ever. "I hear you've got a princess in your house," the callers say. "Congratulations." Julie starts to bask in reflected glory, while Paul is pleased to the point of beatification.

Listening to Carol, I am repeatedly torn. With pride she announces, "I am the first princess ever to have leukemia." And later, in an argument with Les, she states, "Yes, that's all right for you, but I'm not going to live as long as the rest of you are." A bitter self-knowledge drives her; she is ceaselessly on the move. My mind, stuffed with the literary allusions left by several years of graduate studies, reclaims a phrase from the English essayists of the Nineteenth Century, "to burn with a hard gemlike flame." Literature students without exception were accustomed to snicker over this phrase, its *fin de siecle* extravagance. How could I have laughed at these words once? Here, indoors, outdoors, wherever Carol goes, the brilliant flame with its diamond-hard glitter burns and dances before my eyes.

On her seventeenth birthday in November Carol acquires a white mouse which very quickly assumes the status of most favored pet. She neglects Calico who responds with a show of stoical resignation, and pays less attention to Blackie who slinks off and mopes behind the sofa. She no longer wants to be bothered with the aquarium either, and says coaxingly, "Please, Julie, feed my fish for me. I haven't got time any more." Carol explains that she is taking a psychology course and plans to use the white mouse in a special project. She shows me a statement of purpose:

I am going to build a maze and put a mouse in it every day after he is conditioned to a regular feeding time. I will time him and compare his time and also see if there is a plateau in his learning.

Now it seems to me that some precise meaning exists for Carol's sudden preoccupation with the mouse and his maze, if I could only find it. I begin to think of the mouse as an indicator or clue to certain subtle changes in my daughter's behavior. "Mousie, Mousie, Mousie," Carol chants, dandling the sleek creature above the table, fingering the pinkish tail, the alert little head. She lets him agitate the leaves of a foliage plant for a moment, releases him to a ceramic bowl where he rushes about the stalks before being returned to a cage and treadmill wheel. Her father listens to the mouse late at night as it clambers over the turning wheel and has nothing but praise for such a display of energy. "A real worker, that fellow just works hard every minute."

I do not think it is the mouse's energy that captivates Carol, but the creature's peculiar vulnerability. The mouse, conditioned to live without freedom, smallest of the household pets, always excepting the fish, clings to its bars, lies spread-eagled across the cage wires as if it would like to break loose from them, yet is simultaneously embracing their security. Both fragile and tough, the tiny animal has an even more uncertain hold on life than the self-reliant cat or complacent dog. This is how I speculate, watching Carol rub warm white fur tenderly and thoughtfully against her cheek.

From a slender prologue of several pages, Carol's medical file has grown to resemble a heavy volume, one that she is not permitted to read, a stringent hospital rule. This being true, I undergo a sharp thrill of disbelief when I see her pick up the forbidden file from the arm of a chair in the out-patient clinic where it has been abandoned by a forgetful nurse. She reads avidly, refuses to relinquish the volume, saying its contents are rightfully hers. Another nurse who observes Carol and me at odds, friction in the air, prises the file from Carol's hands and carries it off as if she were retrieving a document of state.

"Acute myeloblastic leukemia.... in remission *now.*" Irony underscores her tones. "Did I ever tell you, mother, that future leukemia cures—well, there aren't any. There will only be vaccines—preventative. Nothing else. They won't be able to cure me." She is looking deep within herself. "Nothing can save me." The words resonate, bounced off from the stone walls of a shaft down which she is peering and examining a terrifying spacelessness.

"Oh, yes, something can." I kiss her unsteadily, I, the mother-become-priestess. "The power of healing will, love and faith, the Holy Spirit." I believe each word and command my belief to pour into Carol like fresh spring water.

After this episode, seemingly minor, I notice and record further change in Carol, a new independence and assertiveness, below which lurk an ever-present irony and self-knowledge. The dancing flame burns more unflinchingly than ever.

It is I who flinch and falter. On some days I am so

possessed by love and pain, freshly wounded and unable to staunch the wound, that I long for a disguise to cover me. I go to the Charismatics and seek the refuge of strange languages, pray in tongues, a river of sounds, spontaneous, with the inflections of ancient or modern European speech dropping from my lips. At other times I write for hours or meditate in silence. I respond constantly to the rhythms of music and swimming; without any particular preliminary summons these rhythms are capable of inducing the presence of the quicksilver image who comforts me and adds her strength to mine.

One afternoon Carol, cuddling her mouse and letting it wander freely along her arm, tells us, as if introducing an after-thought, that several boys have been calling her up and she is no longer going to spend her time with Steve exclusively. "I'm playing the field from now on," she says coolly. The mouse crosses over and sits on one of her shoulder blades including us all in its dark-focused enigmatic view. "Mother, don't tell me how unfair I am," Carol explodes before I can open my mouth. "I'm going to be free and unattached in the future. I don't need any boy friend!"

She informs her fascinated audience, furthermore, that three boys want to take her out Saturday night. She smokes a cigarette moodily, as if expecting an argument.

"If you're not seeing Steve this weekend, then which one of the—who would your date be?" I ask.

"Maybe all three of them," she retorts, studying the expression on our faces with amusement.

It is all bluff. She doesn't mean it. She spends the entire weekend with Debbie and Les, her oldest friends.

Chapter 22

The first reference to a bone marrow transplant. Paul listens to a radio interview with a San Francisco doctor who has just used this revolutionary new surgical technique. The operation involved a pair of twins, one as patient, the other as donor. The surgeon remarks, "The life expectancy of an acute leukemia patient is normally from three to four years." His statement infuriates Paul who expects modern medicine and the ministrations of the City of Hope to cure Carol.

We debate the transplant technique, the broadcast, our own mixed feelings. In my opinion, I comment, it is futile to get angry over the public pronouncements of a surgeon; but my words just refuel Paul's indignation. On this same day I attend a church service where I hear an Episcopalian nun commend the spiritual benefits of absolute silence and withdrawal; she goes further and speaks of the obligation every person has, "to yield and give...not an erasing of identity, but a reliance upon God with an expectant trust in what God does with one's life."

The nun has defined faith. My feelings become even more complicated before the obvious sincerity and ardor of her private vision. That haunted corner of my brain where the murmex-critic broods now examines meaning carefully, redefines and reproaches an inappropriate passivity. The nun has no child, murmex points out, she protects herself from desperation and fear, she is not skirmishing with Leukos the destroyer. Withdrawal to a mountain retreat may be exactly right for her, but not for you. Do not yield to passiveness or to the destroyer; do not submit. Think of Tolkien's fellowship of the ring, the heroic endeavor. But I am no hero, I protest, and I have no loyal companionship. I am alone.

As if to contradict me, friends materialize. Barbara and Sue drop in, Michele phones from Hollywood, Lenore assures me that she and many other Charismatics are praying for Carol's complete recovery. "With God anything is possible," she affirms. I ought to feel better, but instead I find myself floundering, sinking to my knees, weeping in corners. *Stop this*, I command to my diary, *overcome anxiety, think what it is like for her.* My pen goes out of control: *Let her live, only let her live and live and live and live and be well.*

December is upon us all at once. Dr. Graham returns. Carol, who has become attached to Dr. Kellon and his easy-going manner, asks me forthwith: "Mother, I want to keep Dr. K. for my doctor. Will you help me?" I broach the subject to Dr. Graham as soon as it is feasible, aware that she does not like the idea much. She frowns, hesitates, then acts briskly impersonal. "Well, this sometimes happens, naturally...but of course, it can be done." The transfer is accomplished.

Carol decides to make her own gifts for the holidays. The kitchen grows aromatic, tinged with lemon and honey, as she dips cherries and pineapple, almonds and walnuts, in pans of hot bubbling light or dark chocolate, and sets the rich confections on wax paper to harden. She carries a large box garnished in scarlet ribbons to the nursing station at the City of Hope. The nurses and aides swarm around her, sampling chocolate and orange peel, exclaiming, "Oh, Carol, thanks... How great you look!"—a refrain repeated by the young man who used to wheel her solicitously from Admissions to her room in Wing Five. "See, Carol, I knew you'd do good. I just knew it," he says. Warmed by the glow of the faces grouped about my daughter, I absorb the moment, the now of time, likening it to a soft candy and sinking into the juicy center gradually, prolonging the savor.

Past and present are interwoven when the winter holiday brings our family of five back together again. We celebrate in the accustomed manner by taking a harbor cruise aboard the Chipsee. A nostalgic day, spiced with memories, some explosions of joy, a few tears. Amy and Carol are both older and have gone through many changes.

"Gosh, Amy, you've gotten taller," Carol says.

"Yeah, Carol, and you've gotten prettier," Amy answers, but the real changes go unmentioned.

The Chipsee sweeps beyond the Queen Mary positioned in Long Beach harbor, passes close to tankers and tug boats and small craft. As in former days when the three daughters were children, Paul lectures, Amy asks questions, Carol and Julie laugh and drowse on the boat cushions. While Carol sleeps, I cup my hands around her toes, feeling the body warmth pulse through a layer of blanket. "Oh God, Holy Spirit, Divinity, whoever you are, help her," I pray. "Strike whatever bargain you want with me, but heal my daughter."

At mid-semester break time, late January, Carol goes to the mountains to share a rented cabin with some of her club friends. A heavy snow falls and they are snowbound; she gets through to me at last by telephone.

"Mother, I've missed the first day of treatment," she says, "and I've been having nightmares."

"You have, Carol?"

"Yes. Nightmares about treatment, bad ones. I don't want to come back, I want to stay here in the snow."

"Oh, darling."

"Mother, mother, I love you."

She returns, dutifully sits in the out-patient clinic, clutching her CBC slip and muttering beneath her breath, "Oh, I hate this, I hate my illness, hate it," saying these words for herself and for me and her father, too, and for every person who loves her.

Kellon confronts Carol. She must be prepared for relapse, he states, because, although the future holds other possibilities, relapse is the most likely occurrence. I look at this word, take it apart. It does not convey any of the personal or philsophical overtones that the term *remission* does, but seems to stand alone, almost without connotations, bleak and stark, self-evident.

Kellon tells me in private, "Oh, recovery is not altogether impossible, a few do actually recover, but the illness is unpredictable and most often our patients go into relapse." Which means, he explains, a new approach. The search begins again for the right combination, and if every treatment fails, death.

Carol says to me, "Well, darn it, if relapse happens, it happens. I just have to go back into the hospital, that's all." She says soberly, "Mother, I'm dying. I have only a little time to live."

Paul is in Europe when these talks with Dr. Kellon occur. I am not able to reach him.

THE SILK OAK TREE

From the beginning it is apparent that the silk oak tree in the front yard is not a climbing tree.

We see the oak for the first time in 1958, when we move to Whittier from our temporary residence in the San Gabriel valley, having lived in California a mere eight months. The tree growing in front of our new home is only a spindly sapling with downswept branches vaguely suggesting the motion of a rotating top. Such branches appear useless to children; they sag, they will not support one's weight like ladder rungs until the climber can reach blue sky. In spite of such an obvious frailty, however, each of the three daughters in time tries to climb the silk oak; each uses her own style, saying little about the effort and giving up quietly in favor of greater rewards proffered by the orange and avocado trees behind the house.

The silk oak grows silently for two decades fulfilling the secret configurations of its invisible seed. Its leaves differentiate into short streamers fluttering from hundreds of tough central ribs, then from thousands, until the tree resembles a huge feather duster swaying in an uncertain wind. Strange clusters of orange flowers form periodically along the limbs. Small brown pods accompany them. Flower and pod drift through the tree like smoke. I have never seen such flowers on a tree before, fringed, almost dripping, and I have never known a tree like the silk oak which grows until its height more than doubles the height of the house.

It will not stop growing. The thousands of leaves become a burden and drag toward the earth. It is a weeping tree with a skinny trunk and a tall crown that promises to obstruct the neighbors' view. The people living behind it will want it topped, I think to myself, watching the amorphous orange flowers weave their fringes into the tapestry of the foliage. The individual leaves are like fans that turn wine-colored several times a year and drop onto the lawn, the hedge and the plants growing in flower pots. There is no end to the work of raking and gathering. We stand on ladders to fish the leaves from the roof, we float them into trash barrels.

Neighbors inform me that the tree's root system must be a vast one, because it has to match the crown, they claim; as much lies below the ground as is seen wavering up above. This is in accordance with the mythology of trees. Those who discourse on the root system also say the tree is a "dirty" one and over-grown, undisciplined. They criticize its stance, its proximity to the house. I am conscious of how much lip service is paid to trees, how human beings profess to love them, but in actuality whenever trees over-state themselves with extensive clutter or sprawl, people cannot wait to take them out.

One night during the windy April month of 1973 as my daughter grows ill and senses changes in her body which she cannot yet openly acknowledge, the silk oak unleashes a single branch close to her window. We are all startled by its size. Carol pulls at the splintered wood. The pupils of her eyes contract until I can see only the soft brown iris, troubled and brooding. "Mother," she says, "I have been dreaming about the tree. It was struck by lightning and fell straight into my bedroom and broke the waterbed. My room flooded, the water kept rising around me—"

I tell her: "Carol, the tree is fine, it's safe, no more branches will drop off" and the ebb and flow of our talking continue—her hesitancy, my reassurance, our interaction establishing a pattern of cross currents that persists through many months.

During the year 1975, the silk oak produces yet another of its unusual manifestations. We are astonished to see streams of resin pour from slight cracks in the trunk. The resin amazes me far more than the exotic fringed flowers; it flows in ropy lengths down the rough bark, a think amber juice collecting insects and particles of cat fur on its way to the ground. The amber substance clutches and droops, glows from brown to gold, is not quite jewel or liquid.

When Carol's veins are lanced at the City of Hope and different fluids are admitted into her body, I can scarcely tolerate the daily presence of the tree's mysterious oozings. To me the tree seems to be emptying its veins, altering its very chemistry, while the life force consolidates and assembles upon the trunk. Unbidden, the tree enters my dreams, suffering, or so my intuition perceives, from such a loss of energy that transfusions are necessary. The silk oak is surrounded by metal poles and plastic bags that drip slowly into the crevices that punctuate its bark. This dream returns even after the cracks in the living tree seal themselves and the rich brown effusions cease to flow.

Changes occur. Without warning a leakage develops across the sidewalk in front of the house. The leak lies directly below the tree, at the foot of the sloping yard and a broad swath of ivy. Some pipe in the ground has broken; this is how we reason. We study the tree, try to predict when the dark fluids will pour over the sidewalk, intermittently staining the pink clover in the parkway. Slowly the clover deteriorates. Encrustations of green slime establish themselves, a dank smell permeates the air above the sidewalk, hosts of tiny gnats appear.

Before long a boy in the neighborhood slips on the slime, but is fortunately uninjured. What repairs must be made, where does the responsibility lie? we ask.

The city authorities come to investigate these issues. They announce that the break in the underground network of pipes occurs within our property line and is therefore our responsibility. The city has nothing to do with over-seeing repairs or paying for them; but it advocates immediate action on the part of the landowners.

We analyze the front lawn, locate the hypothetical break at some point beneath the tree's exploring roots. The tree is guilty, the tree must be removed. People suggest it could unleash more disasters and threatens us from top to bottom. We decide to do away with this menace; and a very long process starts, the removal of the tree.

A professional tree service begins. It sends a team of lumber-jacks to saw and cut and pare until only the central trunk is left projecting eight feet above ground like the mast of a ship. The professionals depart. We, all of us, hoist shovels and dig a trench around the stump. We carve out a trough which gradually grows wider and deeper. Neighbors, even a few strangers, come into the yard, drawn by the sight of the desiccated stump or by an impulse of curiosity. They make jokes, see the trough as a wading pond, the dog's bathtub and the like. We fill the pit with water from the hose to soften the ground for digging and watch the slowly emerging root pattern.

A chain hoist is brought in and securely linked from the stump to a telephone pole in the parkway. Boards are laid down. We stand on them, take our turns pulling at the hoist. After a few hours the mechanism is shifted from the telephone pole to a neighboring sycamore. We continue pulling, tug with bare hands at the heavy chains, hearing behind us the groans and cracking explosions made by the tree as it is sucked from the earth. Protesting and lamenting, the silk oak lifts out, crashes on its side above the bank of ivy.

The tree's entire subterranean structure is laid bare to us. The roots radiate from the center, keep to the horizontal, reminding me of an accordion pleat. They bear no resemblance to the top of the silk oak at all, as the myth insists, but ramble off at right angles, each root choosing its own shape and path to nourishment. These roots have never grazed a pipe, have never even come close to destroying anything. Somewhat dazed, we peer into the crater left by the tree and see the pink clay sewer pipes, see the breaks in them, the damaged joints made, not by the silk oak, but by some unknown motion of the earth. A tremor that occurred years ago, an earthquake, we murmur, *of course;* and automatically we begin to replace the pipes, replace the soil, filling in and returning whatever we have taken out.

Before much time has passed, we stop, immobilized, unable to complete the work because of a flaming furious red rash that breaks out over everyone's hands and wrists. The rash cannot be contained but proceeds to spread leaping on our bodies like a forest fire. "What is wrong?" we ask each other in bewilderment. "The tree is a silk oak, not a poison oak," we protest, unable to explain so much discomfort. What forces are being released here? I wonder to myself. How is it that none of us has ever actually understood this tree?

We summon other people to finish chopping up the stump and roots, ask them to carry the logs away. When the last log is removed and our torment has been forgotten, we begin to consider the virtues of the tree that is no longer there. We remember its odd beauty, the surprises that were so often revealed to us: the floating diaphanous orange flowers, the masses of delicate leaves, the birds that settled in the top branches and flew to Carol's window ledge to be fed from a wooden tray. We recall the gracefulness, the movement, the stature and brilliance of this remarkable tree.

How peculiar it all is, I say, and start to sow fresh seed across the lawn. The harsh glint of the sun upon my daughter's bedroom windows causes me to hesitate; I enter the house, thinking to close these windows and protect the walls and carpeting from the glare.

Carol's room seems to be baking. It gives off heat like a forge, is filled with the violence of flame. Heat pours in through the glass panes, swirls in torrents past the flowered curtains. There is nothing to hold it back. The tree is gone.

Chapter 23

Valentine's Day. Paul is going to broil steaks for us tonight. I give all three daughters gingerbread hearts and slim gold rings with tiny chip diamonds in them—guard rings, I call them.

"Well, everybody," Paul says, removing the steaks from the broiler. "I have an announcement to make. Are you ready?"

"Sure, dad," Julie answers. "What's the surprise?"

"I've been promoted," he says proudly. "The corporation has, well—let's put it this way—a couple of other plants are going to report to me from now on." He beams.

We exclaim in unison and congratulate him. Carol stares at her steak. I can see it is too rare for her and put it back on the broiler. "Where else will you be travelling, daddy?" she asks.

"Oh, Tennessee and Ohio."

"And New York state, too?"

"Uh huh. That's right." He does not have to mention Europe or the fact that his trips abroad are redoubling in frequency.

Carol flings her arms around Paul and begins to joke. Julie asks, "Gosh, dad, when can I go to Italy?" Amy says, "But will you still coach me for my interview next week?" She is living in an apartment in east Whittier and applying for job interviews. My mind a turmoil, I try to equalize two facts: Paul receives a promotion, Carol is warned about relapse. The two statements see-saw, up and down, out of balance. The dinner ends and I question him privately. "Can you remember Carol last year at this time? How we raced to the basketball court in the gym, remember the pink dress she made, her rose, how healthy she looked then?"

"Yes, sure, of course I do," he says gruffly. He does not want to sound sentimental even on Valentine's Day. I fantasize him briefly as an ambassador, a man with a portfolio who will never stop for long in any one place again or set his portfolio down to rest. The first fine vibrations of profound change electrify the room. I discern the future breaking out of its chrysalis and intuit that from now on I, too, like the manufacturing plants in Milan and Knoxville, will be making periodic reports to Paul.

He asks me who Carol's current boy friend is.

"It's Ron," I state. "She's been seeing him a lot."

"The boy with the dark hair and eyes, white teeth, what does he do?"

"He's athletic, he skiis and plays baseball. Works hard, too."

"Carol likes a do-er."

"Ron makes her laugh and he thinks.... He says she's going to get well."

Our eyes meet. "She keeps asking me," I say steadily, "'Mother, will I die of this? Mother, where is the cure?' *Well, where is it?*" I blaze.

"Yes. Where." The furrows arrange themselves on Paul's forehead. "A bone marrow transplant? That might be the answer."

Shortly before the next treatment I take part in a poetry reading at Laguna. A good many women attend, old friends I haven't seen for a while because of my involvement with the Charismatics and other groups. The next day I accompany Carol to the out-patient clinic. Kellon studies her latest CBC slip, regards me obliquely before saying, "Her counts are still within the normal range. We'll go on as usual."

I drive home a bit absent-mindedly. "Mother, concentrate, will you, please, on your driving?" Carol scolds, reproving me as she has not done since last summer. She rushes into the house and vomits over the bathroom floor. Dazed, clutching the molding of the doorway, she apologizes: "I'm so sorry, mom, I'm so sorry, sorry!"

I can scarcely bear her abjectness, the humility. Tension climbs inside me like root sap ascending the crown of a tree, passing from one wood cell to another. The tension makes it futile for me to go to the scheduled Monday evening prayer group. I feel my anxieties would be interpreted as weakness which in turn would be translated as a lack of faith. Spoken or unspoken, this accusation is one I cannot tolerate just now.

I stay at home. I meet Leukos alone, on his own terms. It is his wish to be met and to be understood, he explains. No matter how analyzed and described by theologians, thinkers, writers, artists, whether seen as white or black or scarlet, horned or winged, Leukos considers himself under-valued and misunderstood. He is able to convey this thought to me and much more.

His embrace blends passion and zeal, an absolutism that keeps me close as an eyelash welded to an eyelid, closer, I live within the expanding pupil of despair. He beguiles and reassures. Leukos would like to be my friend. The lonely terrain on which our tryst takes place has room for no other being, he says; he will be my world.

I am a swimmer, I tell him, I am not bound to his terrain, but to the living water—the seas, the lakes and rivers and, by extension, to all that is fluid as well, to rhythms, melody, color. I evoke music as an ally, whispering defiance to Leukos, my voice dropping to a chant. The small radio under my hand unleashes a volume of melody that sweeps us apart: fast, faster, breath and movement, the singing, the reaching, music and rhythm one. He no longer holds me rigid and close to his dry skin, bemused by the orbs of his white eyes. He will never entrance me again. I swim forth, free.

But I am not alone. As Leukos diminishes, a wheel is turned, the Companion evolves, although not by my summons or conscious wish. Out of the depths of sound her mercurial image is borne. I name her the Comforter and the Companion. Through our communication anguish and meaning both flow, the knowledge that I am part of a vast linkage to every other form, each manifestation of life, and to death as well—the shapes of the blackbird as it flies, fruit ripening, the decayed stump, ashes, flesh, foam, and, my anguish speaks, to Carol's changing courses, whether they wax or wane.

With the Charismatics throughout the passing weeks I explore the intricacies and improvisations of ecstatic sound, glossalalia; but this is by no means all. Mystery and ecstasy do not remain the central focus. Emphasis shifts; it moves to study groups and intellectual discussions, to, at last, human morality. The chastening indictment of the sins of the flesh, guilt, the condemnations, the anger of the evangelist Paul are exactly as I remember them, not one whit softened. The weaponry of sin, fixed and catalogued in Paul's writings, is exposed in a fury of words. I re-read the catalogue: lust, greed, malice, murder, deceit, hate, disobedience, insolence, lying. I put the list aside because it wearies my spirit, it is of no use to me or to Carol. As for the heavy whiplash of sin and guilt, I seize it by the handle and hurtle it through the air.

Chapter 24

Carol corners me while I hang a dripping swim suit next to a cap and a pair of goggles on the clothesline. She catches a few drops on one palm and looks up into my face challengingly. "Mother, why won't you ever talk to Ron?" she demands.

"I'll be glad to, honey," I reply, "if you want me to. You just have to bring him around more often. How about this afternoon?"

She brightens, drapes a wet towel over the line for me. "Mom, I didn't tell you yet, but one of the nurses, it wasn't Birdie or Cathy Robinson or any of those we know—well, anyway, this one said, 'Carol, you're really an amazing gal. Your count is higher today than it was yesterday.' She told me that Dr. Kellon is even impressed by my performance."

"She said that? Well, how good, Carol." I give her a hug but my mind has taken another leap into speculation and perplexity. Why is illness regarded as a form of competition, why is Carol supposed to be in competition with herself? I can't slow down my thoughts or avoid certain jarring conclusions: as long as the blood counts are good or within the acceptable range, she will be praised; if they deteriorate, she can expect disapproval from both nurses and doctors; relapse must mean the height of failure then. My church friends' interpretation will be, covertly, of course, failure, loss of faith, guilt. Yes, guilt forever sticks, the palimpsest is never quite scraped clean; and these days I am never very far away from the memory and sound of the tent evangelist's wrathful blaming voice.

The bitterness of these reflections follows me through the day. I cannot shake it off. When Ron arrives at the front door, a little unsure of himself, we greet each other with smiles and pleasantries, but I am not up to a sustained conversation. I take refuge in chiding Blackie who is rolling happily on the rug. Carol and Ron lead the dog outside. I brush apple cores and carrot tops from the kitchen counter, my thought still focused ironically upon the race Carol runs and runs in the acute leukemia event.

During March Carol thinks she sees signs of relapse. She quarrels with Ron and with Debbie and then rages at me: "I'd like to hate you, mother, I really want to hate you, but I just can't."

"Go ahead, Carol, if it helps."

She addresses her older sister, "Amy, listen, I may have to try a different treatment soon."

"Yes, Carol?" Amy frowns.

"And one kind of treatment, well, it makes you really fat."

"Yeah. I guess you don't want that, do you?"

"And another sort makes you bald."

"That's not so bad. Y'know, I'm selling wigs now in the accessory department at the store and I can set some aside for you to try on if you want me to."

Carol smiles. Her anxiety is curbed one moment, rampaging the next. Just before driving to school she discovers that she has a sore throat and gives herself an antibiotic. I panic, telephone Paul at his office, call my friend Joyce, and the City of Hope in rapid succession. A nurse promises to order more antibiotic and soothes: "We'll be seeing her Monday for a check-up and I'm certain she'll be all right in the meantime..."

As the emotional tides rise higher Mr. Small telephones.

"Her blood count has been fluctuating wildly for days," I tell him.

"Mary, think positively, only positively," he says with firmness. "It is important not to take the attitude the world does. The world looks at the medical diagnosis and thinks of just one path—downhill. But we don't believe that. We have faith and we can remove mountains."

"Oh, I do, too, I have faith," I say choking, the tears thick in my throat.

"No one can be as close to Carol as you are," Mr. Small says sympathetically. "That is hard, a difficult position to be in. But do remember that we are all praying for her."

Minutes later Joyce comes down the hill bringing a copy of *The Princess* with her, a book by a Finnish writer that describes the author's marriage to a young nurse afflicted with Hodgkin's Disease and undergoing radiation treatments. The woman's intense will to live and her determination to bear a child in spite of the odds somehow propel her into a remission that appears to be permanent. It is a vibrant story and one I hope to see repeated, I tell Joyce.

"Yes, dear, love can do wonders," Joyce affirms.

I hear a different message, however, from yet another friend who calls and states bluntly, "Mary, she's going to die. Face reality."

In this welter of conflicting advice and ambiguous consolation I concentrate upon the reality of Carol herself, her presence, the unmistakable fact that now, today, she remains alive.

Kathryn Kuhlman, who has an international reputation as a faith healer, comes to the Shrine Auditorium in Los Angeles in April to conduct a healing service. Carol agrees to attend. Prior to the event I write the evangelist and request that she pray for my daughter; the response from the Kuhlman Foundation, while considerate and positive, states that the healer does not pray for individuals at the Shrine, but offers a general petition to God which is usually of benefit to members of the audience.

Carol and I board a crowded bus on a drizzling wet morning, stand in a line that winds across several sidewalks, squeeze into two seats high above a big brilliantly lighted stage. The choir hums and sways, filled with men in blue suits and women wearing bright chiffon gowns, pink, purple, orange, wildflowers seen from a distance stemming a prairie wind. They sing and ripple, briskly, dramatically. Kathryn Kuhlman extends the drama, dazzles, clad in pure white, her motion almost dancelike. She projects charm, humor, personal magnetism and something else, a quality no one can really put into words, a power of a sort that causes a great many men and women to throw down crutches and braces, abandon their wheelchairs, and stumble over the stage in tears, declaring their gratitude to God.

Unobtrusively I consider my daughter's reactions to this emotional performance and see that before long she applauds and sings and prays when everyone else does; but that her eyes stray occasionally from the lighted platform to study the faces and forms of the people in the audience. When the service ends after three hours, we cannot leave the building right away; the aisles are blocked with wheelchairs and crippled folk. Carol glances to the right and left, "Oh, my goodness." She sighs and speaks in a subdued whisper that is meant for my ears only. "I'm not so bad off, after all, mother. These poor people are the ones who really need help, aren't they?"

DAFFODIL, ASPHODEL

"What's an asphodel?" Carol asks me one morning. She is twelve years old, puzzling over a homework assignment in a mythology book.

"Oh, it's a flower," I reply and then, being pressed further, I tell her what I can remember and consult an encyclopedia for more information about this mysterious plant.

The ancient Greeks, I read, regarded the silvery asphodel as the flower of the dead. Its habitat was the Elysian fields, those vague and shadowed meadows that antiquity placed either underground or upon low-set islands of the western ocean.

"But are there any asphodels today?" Carol wants to know and to satisfy that inquiry I read on and discover that two flowers by the name of asphodel, one yellow and the other white, still grow around the Mediterranean basin. "The spring daffodil, beloved by the western Romantic poets of the Nineteenth Century, derives from this legendary blossom," I read aloud from my source book, "the term daffodil being a corruption of the true name asphodel."

There is a prolonged silence. "Daffodil?" Carol asks. "You mean that isn't its real name, you mean it's honestly something called an *asphodel*?"

I admit that the book says this is so.

"I really like daffodils," Carol says impulsively. "Why don't we ever have any in our garden?"

I do not want to acknowledge that, after more than a decade of living on the west coast, I am still accustoming myself to its unfamiliar flora, plants like hibiscus and cactus and camellia, and am not yet certain which midwestern flowers do well in the arid climate of southern California. "The bulbs are very bitter," I answer, "and your cat might eat them."

Carol hoots at me.

I mollify her a little by describing the wild daffodils that climb up the steep bluffs ringing Lake Michigan and infiltrate the parks and lawns of Milwaukee; I mention the golden trumpet variety that used to dominate the borders of my mother's spring garden and Carol and I discuss planting some daffodils at a future date, along with complementary bulbs of narcissus and hyacinth.

Four years after we hold this conversation flowers of all varieties become a vital presence in our lives. People carry bouquets and potted plants, single sprays and clusters, to Carol at the hospital or at home. They give her roses and carnations, camellias, azaleas, daisies, chrysanthemums, cornflowers, iris, gardenias, cyclamen, dahlias, circled by a corona of ferns or leaves or delicately filigreed with white baby's breath.

During the passing months I learn that the significance of flowers is by no means limited to the positive act of giving. Flowers convey message and nuance. Mediaeval overtones filter from the whorled centers and textures of the petals, from the variegated colors, the clear pinks and lavenders, the warm shades and the cool. With the different fragrances I imbibe a sense of the flower as symbol and meditation image, its power as a healing talisman.

Occasionally someone brings daffodils to Carol. "See, mother," she says, detaching a ruffled blossom from its setting and stroking the orange-rimmed cup. "Look. My favorite colors are in this flower, yellow and orange. I think daffodils must be my favorite flower, too..."

One March day while Carol is undergoing chemotherapy I come upon a stall where daffodils are being sold at an open-air market in Hollywood and I bring yellow and white clusters of them to her at the City of Hope.

She is sleeping when I walk into her room, so I fill the vases, placing the flowers upon a tray alongside the bed and step back a few paces into a hazy rectangle of sunlight that streams through an uncurtained window. Carol's sleep is profound, her breathing deep and even. A wind outside blows and blows against the branches of a tree which is beginning to leaf into spring green; the wind's pulsations seem timed to correspond with Carol's own deep breaths. For a few minutes I enter the same rhythmical continuum that embraces my daughter and the wind outside, my breath rising and falling as theirs does; just so long I experience a subtle happiness, I feel myself at the very center of some limitless and sustaining energy.

Carol wakes up. She smiles and touches the daffodils. "Thank you, mother," she says. "I want you to take some with you when you go back home." She assembles a bouquet which later occupies a vase on my dresser and fills the room with fragrance.

I think about the daffodils and meditate upon their gold-tissue throats which lean toward me as if to utter a confidence. I notice how they are fashioned, the two distinctive elements, the aureole of petals or perianth and the full trumpet, which, in other varieties is also called the cup or crown or eye. And it follows, then, that the daffodil is actually more than flower, being both trumpet and eye, speaking and seeing, a visionary oracular plant.

Near the edge of the golden bouquet that Carol has given me one small white blossom shimmers. I look long at the eye of this single flower. Its paleness grows paler, the white hue more white. Within the crown of living petals the asphodel opens its silver bloom.

Chapter 25

It is May, almost a year to the day when Carol first learned of her illness. Dr. Kellon tells me she is now in relapse.

He takes me into his office and talks about the bone marrow test he has just run. He is stern, rather curt, no longer the amiable doctor, but the seer with a painful vision to impart. As I leave his office, numb and unspeaking, Carol steps out from the wall and assumes a brisk verbal offensive. "I heard what he said, mother," she says accusingly. "You might as well tell me everything. I already know the worst."

That this is not true, that she is tricking me, inventing, I am too distraught to perceive at once. "He thinks...the bone marrow...results," I blurt, taken off guard, "...then you heard him say you might have to go back into the hospital soon..."

She begins to cry softly.

Kellon is troubled by this bit of drama and turns Carol over to me exclusively. It is I who must quote the doctor, saying, "You are not in great immediate difficulty, but the test reveals you have become 'cellular'; that, once more the immature white cells are present, the white count and the hemoglobin are down too far. Not remission anymore, he says, but relapse."

"Ah, mother, I realize it," she says at last. "I know something is wrong. There's a strange ache in my mouth and

I can feel the difference in my blood."

Kellon has already told me what his procedure will be. He intends to increase the frequency of the present chemotherapy, applying it every two weeks in an effort to force the count up. This he will attempt at least three times. If the count does not rise, he will re-admit her to the hospital and the search for a successful form of treatment will continue.

Paul, who has just returned from Italy, is as stunned as I am. At first he refuses to believe the news, blusters, demands to see Kellon himself and look at the slides. He talks to Kellon, comes home shaken.

I make phone calls to the Monday night group and to my sister, who says that she and her husband will fly to California next month in order to attend Carol's high school graduation. I have thought little about graduation lately, I tell her, but please come.

The need for action possesses me; at the same time I feel crippled by paralysis. I write letters, puzzle over composing sentences in my diary, swim, walk idly to the top of the hill's second hump; coming down, I thrust my hands into clumps of tropical plants, odd formations I do not know the names of, bitter aloe, perhaps, I muse, and turn the fleshy leaves aside, as if I were looking for something, a fruit, a promise. Carol is also going through motions, playing tennis, cutting out a long dress to sew for the senior prom, putting the pieces of a complicated jigsaw puzzle together. Suddenly every one of us comes down with the flu. I enter a region of white staring spaces and gray shadows, emptiness and estrangement.

But I am well enough when the time comes for Carol to go to the City of Hope. After treatment, as we walk under trellises and alongside flower beds refulgent with soft bloom, leaving the out-patient clinic and its paraphernalia behind, a feeling of complete unreality grips me. We have done all this before. Were the events of last summer, then, no more than a dress rehearsal? The rehearsal is done, finished. Are we about to take part in the real action?

The part my daughter plays is one she has no difficulty

remembering: the severe nausea, the appearance of malaise, the drift into semi-consciousness. Blackie knows his role, too, once again the ferocious protective guard who will not let me approach his mistress and limits me to the margins of her room. Hypnotized, the attendant who recalls, but no longer understands, her function, I wait at the threshold until I am almost bereft of thought. Her face occupies me. I gaze, I believe I have never seen a face like hers before, marked by starker, more poignant lines.

She keeps a copy of the Bible and Kathryn Kuhlman's book, *I Believe in Miracles,* beside her; the slender fingers rest gently on the book cover. Images of the healing service we attended last month saturate my mind—the joyful recoveries, people made whole again.

I summon my resources—prayer, more prayer as an adjunct to treatment. Away from Carol's languor, the stunned aftermath of chemotherapy, I fall to the floor, kneel. Is this the posture God prefers? My hands plead. Perhaps Deity is growing tired of hearing from me so often. Please, is God listening?

Chapter 26

Carol cuts her hair short. The straight yellow strands swing loosely about her face, veiling the bruise on her cheek, the blue-black mark left by a carelessly opened refrigerator door. She tans herself resolutely beneath the sun-lamp while one foot taps at an oily rag and several cardboard color samples dropped on the living room rug. A tenacious silence has been hanging over the room ever since the painters' departure.

"How soon are they going to get the paint job finished, do you think?" she asks me at last. "Is it going to be in time for my graduation or not?"

"It had better be," I say. "Your aunt and uncle are due to arrive in a couple of weeks. It's got to be done by then."

She frowns up into the ceiling. "Well, I'm glad they're coming, but I'd better warn you, I won't be around much after graduation. I'm going on a trip to the Colorado river: a bunch of us, I mean, are going down for three whole days. It's just the seniors this time."

I ponder this information. It will not be her first river trip and I know what to expect. "I suppose you'll be wanting to drive the Monte Carlo, then, won't you?"

"Oh yes, mom, can I please take it? I've already promised several of my friends, sort of, that I'd pick them up..."

"I see. Well, yes, I think so. Is Les going along, too?"

"Mom, you've forgotten again. Les is in Georgia, remember? She graduated early in January and she's down there with her brother."

"Of course, I did forget."

Silence descends again while I match the paint samples against the walls of the room. The stillness is shattered by an impulsive declaration from Carol: "I talked to Steve yesterday."

"You did? What about?"

"Oh, lots of things. We started out being friendly but then he got all jealous and weird and we had to break it off."

"Carol," I say, changing the subject. "I know how you feel about camping and everything.... but what will you do at the river if the weather gets really hot and muggy? Which it probably will."

The short hair tosses. "Oh, don't worry, we can always find an air-conditioned motel or move in with somebody if we have to. A couple of my friends are renting campers that are pretty neat."

She broods before giving expression to the secret worry that has been bothering her. "Mother, I think there's something the matter with my mouth," she says reluctantly. I drop the paint swatches in alarm. "I can hardly swallow. I think my tongue is beginning to swell up."

It is true. I check her mouth; the muscles cannot hold onto a thermometer. Without pausing to telephone we dash immediately to the City of Hope. Dr. Kellon laughs at us both and explains that Carol's symptoms are merely reactions to compazine, a new nausea pill she has been taking. He prescribes a different medication.

Once at home again and with Carol comforted, I am lightheaded from giddy waves of relief. This won't do, I tell myself. I have not yet found the balance, the mediation, whatever it is, between empathy and objectivity. I am almost never objective any more. The composed nurse and attendant keeping a sensible emotional distance between herself and her charge has vanished, if, in fact, she ever existed. My identification with Carol is simply extending and deepening, part of a process that occurs within an invisible psychic space I inhabit from time to time, but do not control.

Paul's mother telephones from Wisconsin and we talk to her in sequence, sounding falsely bright, like parrots repeating, "fine, fine, everything is fine." The effort of being positive keeps us all wound too tight like violin strings in need of retuning.

Throughout the month of June Carol's blood counts remain in the desired high range. The hospital personnel continue their praise: "Carol, you're doing beautiful! Didn't the doctor tell you?"

"See!" A yellow CBC slip is thrust under my nose. "Look. She's running just a little below average in only a few areas—but the averages we go by are for adults. Now, for a young girl, Carol is doing just great!" Carol sucks on a lemon slice and looks bored.

Perhaps the high count means she will soon be back in remission; how wonderful if this is true. But Kellon offers no real encouragement, only a noncommittal silence. The nurses and aides are the ones challenging and spurring her on. In competition with herself, I muse, what can only be thought of as the race of races, she is performing a good sprint. And for her most recent effort, a reward: no more chemotherapy until after graduation. This laurel is being bestowed with restraint.

In a sense the interval becomes a remission. Carol appears to forget the illness for three weeks. Her happiness echoes like a fine silver bell pealing through the rooms of the house. She sings and chatters and dances from one person to another, restlessness shaping a series of ascending notes played across a chime. She cannot stay still.

"I'm high, mom, I'm high. I can't help it," she chants. "Some of the kids in class even accuse me of being on whites, because of the way I sound all the time now. I can't stop talking. I keep asking questions every day in my classes. But

I'm not showing off; it isn't that, believe me. I'm really and truly interested. I just want to learn as much as I can."

She is still the burning gemlike flame, but at the center of her motion lie an expanding consciousness and zest and sensitivity that are immortal. The impulse to tell her so is strong. Instead, I ask, "What exactly are whites? I mean, naturally they're some kind of pills, I understand that, a drug of some sort—"

"They're uppers," she replies. "And they eat up the white cells in a person's body. That's why they're called 'whites.' You know darned well I would never take anything like that! But other girls take them sometimes to reduce. Yes, they really do."

"Incredible." The word is shopworn, but it is the only one that will suffice.

After my sister and brother-in-law arrive, I write very little in the diary, except for a sketchy attempt to describe the heat, the odd casual dreamlike quality of graduation day; I quote the student speaker who, in a burst of enthusiasm for "scientific achievement" mentions the "progress being made in over-coming leukemia." Carol raises her eye-brows. "Why say that?" she demands fiercely.

She is ready to take flight. Phil's camera catches one fleeting instant of time, then another: Carol wearing a burgundy cap and gown; in a short pink dress standing next to her father outside his shop door; surrounded by her sisters; at the wheel of the Monte Carlo.

Barely able to control her excitement, looking pinker by the moment, almost the color of a rosy peach, Carol leaves for the Colorado river. Bea and Phil take me aside. Together they ask, "Is she really in relapse?"

"Yes."

"Well, could the doctors possibly be wrong?"

Chapter 27

Dr. Kellon is smiling at Carol who has just bombarded him with a volley of questions. "But, listen to me, Dr. Kellon, I'm really serious. What's going to happen? Am I going to gain weight or lose all my hair or just what?" she repeats anxiously.

He laughs. An impression of strong white teeth in a black pleasant face, the elevation of a grizzled beard. "Now, now, Carol, if we change treatment, you won't have any more reactions to deal with than what you do today"—referring, of course, to nausea.

Carol, thin and rather nervous, looks at him with an exasperation that gradually lessens as the doctor continues to cajole and joke. Her melancholy subsides.

Flowers from Ron are waiting for her at the house. She inhales their scent, picks a few shattered rose petals up from the floor and says, "Well, whenever they do find a cure, it'll be too late for me."

A sudden physical wrench takes place inside of me at these words, as if every organ in my body had lurched out of position. I struggle to re-arrange myself, masquerading, searching for her new nausea medication, the tigan. The rest of the evening a stern-faced Carol cuts out and sews a light-weight robe, vomiting repeatedly, but finishing the robe.

Midsummer, a time for vacation and travel. Paul goes to the east coast. Dr. Kellon takes two weeks off. Carol and Julie, along with a complement of their friends—Debbie, Tracy, Susan—rent a cottage at Newport Beach. Carol has exacted a promise from Kellon that no more chemotherapy will be scheduled until August 20. She is exhilarated; the days turn golden again.

Amy and I keep in touch. Still, there is no denying that the house has emptied once more and silence sifts from the hillside down through the half-opened windows, broken only by the outcries of the cats, the barking dog, the whirling of the mouse treading the wheel of its cage.

The quiet exudes a rare balm. I have no wish to leave. Even if I wanted to travel somewhere, I could not possibly go. My legs have betrayed me; the veins I have been trying to ignore are inflamed, phlebitis, my doctor insists, further aggravated by a muscle spasm of the right hip. He urges surgery, vein-stripping. I put him off and settle into a state of immobilization.

I give up swimming. The Monday night group meets less frequently during July and August; my contact with other people diminishes. I separate from the Charismatics, writing to the rector and explaining that it has become impossible for me to maintain my current schedule; the driving alone is prohibitive. For the Charismatics' prayers and support, my heartfelt thanks. I hope the congregation will continue to sustain Carol in their thoughts.

I make no reference to the study groups and their intellectual content which forces me into periodic confrontation with the evangelist Paul. Intuitively I seek relief from the evangelist's vocabulary of human error and shame, the dichotomies of sin and atonement. As for the ability to speak and sing in tongues, if this is a true transcendence, I believe it will succor me regardless of my surroundings.

Summer is at low tide. With both legs bandaged and elevated as much as possible, lying horizontal on bed or floor, I write poetry and a commentary in my diary that roams from dialogue to argument into an examination of the meanings of words. I look at the sounds I call *core words,* those resting at the center of things like seeds or essences, the groupings of Greek and Latin syllables that were molded into verbs and nouns in the southern peninsulas of Europe and were later borne north to the forests of France and Saxony where they encapsulated further meanings. For me the core words, the seeds, have a fragile complexity, a radiance and tenderness that other words lack. I consider a few of them: courage, endurance, love and the sacred. These words matter, have always mattered.

Love. The Anglo Saxon root is *lufu* and it is akin to a word that means "to believe." Almost endless definition and nuance imbue the term, but what does it mean to me now, during this slow waning summer?

I choose a metaphor. Love: a conflagration, a state of being consumed. Within myself a kind of liquid lava burns, has burned, is burning, ever so surely, tissue by tissue, the soft interior portions, the lungs, brain, heart, pancreas, spleen, and beyond all these the hard implacable substances of the ego. This fiery love is not focused exclusively upon Carol or the other members of my family. Like Phlegethon, the mythological river of fire, it rushes forward at times to encircle whatever settles in its path. It flickers and plays across every sort of artifact and creature. Boundaries crumple, fold. I close my eyes and am invaded immediately by a montage of remembered beauty: high seas rolling past; sandpipers, as I have often seen them, poking their thin beaks into the surf; the crystalline face of a rocky ledge split by an upheaval of the earth; the green spears thronging a grove of bamboo; a cloud formation carrying rain in its dense pockets. Whatever I view is worthy of love and reverence.

The sacred: theá, theós. I have ceased to bargain with a divinity who might or might not be kind, who is certainly elusive, and whose alliance with wordly power confuses me. Terms like godhead and ground of being bring me no nearer to deity. Silence, intense listening and concentration, sinking within the layers of my own nature, carry me to sources of both fire and water, into paradox, formlessness, the streaming motion out of which at times the mobile form of the Companion rises. She emerges, a chasm is spanned by her understanding and compassion and strength. Perhaps the Companion is as close as I shall ever come in this life to deity.

When Paul returns from New York, the two of us visit Carol and Julie at the beach. We drive through a maze of tangled streets and tiny houses animated by stereos, guitars and brusque German shepherds. There is no place to park. Paul double-parks. We weave past clothes-lines and fences, find a bridge over a small back-water and, entirely by accident, come face to face with Debbie.

The cottage, which lies just ahead of us, has been cleared of house guests temporarily. Carol and Julie are both enormously proud of their minute quarters, oblivious to inconveniences, wet swim suits, sand and noise. "Awfully close living," I say limping by the windows, aware of the neighbors' scrutiny and the contents of their kitchen shelves. I can read the labels on their cereal boxes, I announce with amusement.

Paul interrogates Carol. "Have you seen Ron lately?" he wants to know. Carol explains that she is tired of quarreling with Ron and now has a new escort named Keith, a student at the University of Utah.

"That reminds me," I say. "A woman from the Admissions office at Rio Hondo called up. I think she wants to talk to you about orientation week."

Carol nods. "It's O.K., I've already found out everything I need to know." A long pause. "I'd better tell both of you. I've decided to sign up for a pre-law course."

"Pre-law?" Paul whistles. "You have, Carol?" He throws up his hands. "Then you've changed your mind again!"

"Sure I have. But you know how much I like to talk. And a lot of people say I'm good at it." Carol gives me a quick glance. "I think mom might like for me to become a lawyer."

"Yes, yes, of course I would," I say.

"Don't worry." Carol is trying to interpret my puzzled

frown. "I know pre-law isn't going to be easy. But I intend to really work."

We stroll out the gate back to the bridge, meeting surfers and sun-bathers and a few fishermen on the way. The sun is setting and lavishing a copper gloss on the stones beneath our feet when we say our goodbyes. The word "treatment" has not been mentioned once.

Kellon, reviewing the latest blood counts. "Platelets are down," he says gravely. "The white count is just too low. Oh, it's not desperately bad, like it was when she first came in here—but it's not good either. She has to organize her education and college classes around her illness."

To me in another aside he remarks, "What she is taking right now is the very best course of treatment available. It is just the best thing we have. I shall abandon it with reluctance."

These statements, brought to Carol's attention, even though softened and phrased somewhat differently, unleash a swift blue moodiness. "Daddy, guess who's still in relapse," she cries out to Paul. "Guess who gets to go back into the hospital for treatment, probably every month from now on!"

"Hey, c'mon, Carol, don't cross that bridge yet." Paul handles her despair in a bluff, half-wry fashion that wins my admiration. The blue eyes and the dark eyes join in one fixed unwavering stare.

"Do you want to see my schedule at Rio this semester?" she asks, suddenly high-spirited, on the up-swing and putting away her desperation.

"Sure I do. Carol, you're going to make a good ambulance-chaser." An exchange of lawyer jokes, low-keyed and ridiculous.

Five days afterward she refuses treatment. *The very first time,* I record in the diary. *I guess it was bound to happen.* And I describe our late arrival at the dim empty out-patient department. Scarcely any attendants are about. A nurse is summoned from a distant wing of the hospital. The strange nurse has difficulty with Carol's veins and after the second failure to find a proper place for an injection Carol folds her arms and declines treatment. "I just want to go home," she announces. A delegation of authoritative personnel arrives. The young Philippino nurse who is friendly with Carol tries to dissuade her.

"No. No treatment," she says firmly. "I'll be coming back in here next week, anyway. It'll be September and the treatment will be changed, I know it will." Head erect, she shakes the tumbled yellow hair. "I'm developing an immunity to this kind. I can feel it. It isn't doing any good. Besides, I don't want to be sick tonight. It seems as if I've been sick for ages. I can hardly remember what it was like down at the beach."

I plead with her, beg, bribe, and grow stern. She refuses. Dr. Fayhe talks to Carol over the inter-hospital phone. "The doctor understands me," she says conclusively. "Now, mother, let's go."

Home again, Carol settles down cheerfully to a large piece of cherry pie.

I sink into torpor, the languid heaviness of the underwater swimmer, who, after the impetus of the surface dive, levels off to enter new streams, the rivers within rivers, colder at every depth and following their own secretive spiralling paths.

Chapter 28

Though I am sitting across the low living room table and at some distance from Carol, I can still recognize her characteristic script sprawled on the single sheet of paper she holds in her hand. From the scratched-out words and doodles curling along the margins I can tell the page is a rough draft.

She doesn't wait for me to make further deductions. "Want to hear what I wrote about myself?" she asks, her manner self-deprecating, features flushed and wearing an air of uncertainty. "I am supposed to describe *me*, in just one page. It's my first assignment in college." She is an upright vivid figure against the green-gold patterns of the couch, all at once as business-like and determined as the crisp corners of her new-bought textbooks.

"That would be for your English class, then," I say.

"Yes, Approaches to Writing, it's called. So, O.K., you're interested, just listen to this." She clears her throat gently; the voice comes out subdued and rather sing-song: "*I am an actress playing the role of Carol Trautmann. From the outside she—the actress—is a typical American teenager. But inside she is more complex, a strong spirit trying to survive.*" She frowns. "Let's skip the next paragraph, I want to work on it some more." A pause, she resumes reading: "*One of Carol's main traits is her curiosity; this aspect is always present in her and has many times caused embarrassment, but mainly it has gained her a wide range of knowledge. She is very interested in human nature."*

"Fine, Carol," I remark.

"Thanks. *Carol is different from many persons her age, for she has leukemia. It is a hard thing to endure sometimes, physically and mentally, but because of her strong will it has never stood in the way of anything she wants to accomplish. The hardest thing about it—*" she rattles the paper emphatically—"*is the way people react to her. She is sensitive to this. But she also enjoys shocking people in many ways, too—*Well, that's as far as I've gotten with it." She tilts her head, regarding me. "You think it's all right?"

"Yes, I certainly do. It's just excellent."

"You do? It is? Good, then." She sparkles with pleasure before plunging into an account of her first week at college, enlivening her talk with imitations of her professors and classmates and, here and there, a glint of satire. The hill at the base of the college is too steep, she says, and the parking lots at the top are too crowded; but she likes her classes, especially Astronomy and tennis. "The Great Religions class, too," she remarks, "but some of the Christians and Jews are already so mad at each other they don't do anything but shout back and forth—and they expect the rest of us to join in." She puts her hands over her ears and shakes her head.

Keith has been escorting her around the campus. "Pretty soon he's going back to Utah," she says, "because he got transferred to the university in Salt Lake City and he's asked me up to visit him for a holiday, maybe. Can I go?"

"I guess you might, but I'm not sure," I say doubtfully.

Carol takes my words to mean an acceptance. She chatters without a break on every subject except chemotherapy until we pull into the parking lot at the City of Hope. Almost visibly she braces herself for a possible change in treatment, but Dr. Kellon changes nothing. He makes a cryptic statement about forcing up the counts and orders the customary cytosine injection and thioguanine tablets. He is grimmer than usual, the nurses more reserved.

When the needle pierces her wrist Carol's eyes become fixed in a rebellious glare. The nurses pretend not to notice; in spite of their tact I receive an overwhelming impression that each one of them is whispering: "See, she's resisting treatment, doing it again, resisting..."

A noticeable difference following chemotherapy: very little nausea, no vomiting. She explains with a certain eager pride, "I'm psyching myself out, just watch me!" and leaves with a group of friends to go dancing in Hollywood. The bravado keeps her going until the next treatment; then, at the moment of injection, she seems to wilt. Seeing her thus one afternoon, forlorn and leaning against the clinic wall, the blunt compassionate nurse named Pat puts her arms around Carol. "It's hell to be sick," she says simply.

Another friendly nurse, Mary Ann, tells me how much she loves my daughter. "Carol's a favorite at this place," she repeats, patting my hand and giving me an anxious look as I wait numbly, a seated caryatid smoothing her features into blank marble.

Carol smiles her bright vivacious smile and finds more friends and new places to dance in Pasadena and Los Angeles. She buys tights and leotards and starts attending a class at a dance studio in Whittier. Les returns from Georgia and the triumvirate of old friends is re-united. There are parties and barbecues and a week-end trip up the coast with Les and Carol taking turns at the wheel and keeping a hilarious diary.

"Les has decided to go to Rio," Carol tells me, "and I didn't think she would, but lots of people we know are signing up for classes, so she thinks she will, too!"

"Lots of people?" I hazard.

"Sure, mom! Sue, Art, Rick, Nadine, Kathy, Linda, Bill, Mike, Yolie...want to hear more?"

I hold up my hands in mock protest.

She is off and away with that furious speed and intensity that keep me fumbling for words. I can only think of fire images and devise a new one to confide to my diary: *The shimmering excitement*, I write, *of an uncontained prairie fire racing through dry grass and sunlight to whatever destiny...*

Fall spins by, emptying its grab-bag of wet days, hot dry spells and orange moons. Carol discovers me one warm evening staring at my legs in a full-length bedroom mirror. I examine the outline of the veins, gingerly test the flow of the blood pushing through them. "My doctor insists that I have surgery for these," I say to Carol. "He claims I can't wait any longer. But, you know, I really don't want surgery. I wish they would just go back in place." I rub at a small ridge. "I guess the valves inside have broken down."

Carol looks at me with sympathy. She hugs me and reveals the red dots forming on her own slender legs, the first ones to appear for many months. In a confidential outburst she admits to an occasional sharp attack of dizziness. Beneath the superficial tan being maintained regularly by the sun-lamp her skin appears tissue-white. A mere day afterward, when the next CBC is analyzed at the City of Hope, Dr. Kellon orders her into the hospital for transfusions. "It's a wonder you haven't fainted on the spot," he says abruptly to Carol, who responds with a clear bright smile.

Kellon calls for a series of treatments to be administered before the transfusions. On the third day of the series Steve visits Carol and I leave them talking together for half an hour while I stroll over to the restaurant and back.

I return carrying a marigold from one of the flower gardens. The atmosphere in the silent room is charged with tension. Steve stares open-eyed at Carol. Carol looks straight ahead of her into the air, as if observing a ghostly pantomime. No needle in sight, no tubing. The I.V. equipment has been pushed to one side. I drop the marigold underfoot.

"What happened?" I ask.

"Dr. Kellon stopped it," Carol says in a constricted voice. "He came in and said my platelet count was down so low this treatment wasn't going to do any good."

Steve swallows. Carol looks at me.

"It's all right, darling," I say quickly.

"After I've been transfused, I'm not supposed to come back here for two whole weeks. And then it's a new try. This time it's for real."

Steve takes a benumbed departure. Carol dawdles over her lunch, withdrawn, refusing to speak until the moment a group of hospital aides enters, in the wake of a young woman—red-haired and slim, holding a bottle of medicine up to one nostril. She makes her unwilling way to the bed next to Carol. Her name is Gayle, she tells us, inhaling the medicine deeply. "Oh, ye gods!" she laments. "I can't believe my platelet count is as low as they say it is. It can't be! I've got a term paper due in ten days!"

She is a freshman at Scripps College in Pomona; the courses she refers to seem to be mainly in the field of literature. She talks distractedly about Shakespeare, the Renaissance, the Sixteenth Century, all the papers she should be writing at this very moment, instead of whiling the time away in a hospital.

"Maybe you can get an extension," Carol says, intrigued by a situation that so closely resembles her own.

"Oh, I already have, believe me. Now I've got to ask for another one," Gayle mourns. "Oh, ye gods! They're going to start my new course of treatment tomorrow. Isn't this a miserable mess? Will you be around here tomorrow, too, Carol?" she asks, a faint ring of hope in her voice.

The sigh I emit, which goes unobserved, is compounded of relief and gratitude. So there is to be some comfort for my daughter in this experience of relapse, a consolation in the form of a new friend, a student her own age, sharing the erratic illness and the unstable future. I think about Gayle and Carol together all the way home and at once describe the new friend to Julie, even before telling her of Dr. Kellon's medical decision.

"He stopped the treatment today," I announce.

"Yes, I thought that would happen," Julie says, taking a loaf of banana bread from the oven. "But Carol's going to be all right, isn't she?"

"Of course she is—will be." I sample the banana bread and go abruptly to my room.

"The treatment has now been stopped," I announce to

the empty rectangle, walls, ceiling and carpet. "Stopped for good." The room is not empty after all, it is not as I left it, but filled with a drifting fog that has floated in through open windows. The weather is changing again from warmth to damp coolness becoming fog. I begin to turn the handles of the levers that operate the windows.

Am I locking the fog inside, or is this possible? Where does the mist go in its circulations? Water is forever going somewhere, always on its way, never arriving, but in the process of movement. Ice into water into fog. Solid to liquid to gas. This heavy mist may travel to the San Bernardino mountains, become snow, drop, become water, a river.... and "the body is a moulded river" the German poet said two hundred years ago...my body, Carol's body, both with their unique circulations; the earth, the winds, the oceans, with theirs. "All will still be well," I repeat to myself. "All is still in process, each of us a part of a larger current. All will still be well," I say, tracing the fog with my hand, laying my fingers lightly across the calves of my legs, hearing the blood shudder, dragging through its channels.

It is Sunday night and Carol remains at home. Paul is in Minnesota. Carol wants to do simple, comfortable things, watch television, bake cookies, cut out a cotton shirt. Working with thread and needle, she smiles at me, not a public medical smile, but one that is genuine and friendly.

Her mood alters. She asks a question: "Mother, am I in worse shape than Gayle? My own platelet count is down to 14,000."

Ah, I reflect, the new friend is also a competitor—Gayle and Carol, participants running the same race, side by side. I say to her: "You are doing all right, Carol. You'll be well. Think of the love around you."

"Mother, am I going to die?"

"No, no, no."

"But the girl I used to see in the out-patient department all the time, the real, real pale one, I think she died, I've not seen her for several weeks."

I am silent, trying to remember the pale girl. I realize that other leukemia patients have died recently; I have overheard Carol and Gayle discussing these deaths in subdued, frightened tones.

"Carol, you have a fine doctor," I say. "The best possible medical help. And lots of spiritual support. Your count is up, this very minute—and you look lovely." I kiss her and wait for my feelings to abate, wanting to do something useful, practical, protective, with the molten churning love that fills me.

Carol senses my turmoil. She talks about lighter subjects and teases her dog, hiding his milk-bones under the sofa cushions. Last week in a private ritual of her own Carol took the white mouse up to the top of the first steep ravine and released the small creature down its plunging sides. "Mousie is gone." She made the announcement as if she had just seen a member of royalty off to the airport. "He is going to mingle with the other field mice and be happy. If a hawk catches him, that will be too bad, but it's better than spending your whole life in a cage."

With the disappearance of the mouse, Blackie and the cats are restored to their earlier prominence. Tonight she feeds her old pets some of the honey cookies she has baked, smears a stiff beauty mask out of egg white over her face, laughs when Blackie fails to recognize her, teases me, cries out: "Mother, mother, I think I am indestructible!"

The next morning she is too tired to get up. She wakes briefly, goes back to sleep, muttering and tossing. Debbie telephones: "Why did you miss English class, Carol?" Les calls next and asks: "Hey, where were you during Government, anyway?" Carol revives, is out of the house and up the hill.

The grace period of two weeks goes by swiftly. In the early moments of the same October day that Carol re-enters the hospital Paul departs on a long journey to Europe. After forty-eight hours have passed, he assures me, he will reach Italy and he will immediately begin rigorous efforts to telephone. His earnest words cannot dispel the lethargy I feel or reduce the chilliness that accompanies me, seeping in from all directions, during the admission procedures at the City of Hope. Alone, I sign the paper authorizing the use of the next new potent drug that will be tried. Azacytidine, it is called. Wordlessly I lay down my pen, my thoughts repetitive, circular. *But I have done this before.* This is an episode within a scene of an act of a play I used to know. Am I in good theatrical form this morning?

Gayle is the first visitor to come into Carol's room, smiling, generous with encouragement and support. She says she is at the hospital for a blood check, nothing more. The woman in the next bed cheerfully confides that her radiation treatment is to begin immediately. The nurses arrive, beaming. Carol jokes with them, smiling her bright medical smile.

I am miles upon the highway beneath dark clouds and wisps of fog before the tight smile on my own face loosens and drops off.

THE RIDE TO HOPE AND BACK

The particular stretch of freeway lying between my house in Whittier, California, and the research center known as the City of Hope is not an ordinary thoroughfare for me. I think of it as the ride to Hope and back, a series of tableaux or vignettes rapidly compressed into forty minutes of driving time.

The drive to Hope begins in the foothills, turns sharply north and encounters at once the cemetery called Rose Hills. My daughter, who sits next to me, her head tilted back, her eyes closed, rests one arm on the car seat. I can see the hand, its tapering fingers and fine nails. My vision expands, I am studying her profile, burning its lines and contours across my mind as if memory were an acetylene torch. I want to remember you forever becomes I want you forever becomes the rhythm of tires rolling over concrete.

The cemetery glitters upon the neighboring slopes, its fences draped with crimson and yellow bloom. One large sign on a high summit enunciates the name ROSE HILLS. My daughter stirs; this is the only time she will ever refer to the cemetery. "Mother," she says, "have you ever thought of Rose Hills?"

My lie is cheerful, emphatic. "No," I breathe, "of course not" and we skim by the Japanese garden with the oval reflecting pool and the dainty bridge which quiver and merge rapidly into the community college. My daughter is a first year student in this very institution but she gives it only a slow measuring glance.

The college rests on its own hilltop like a guardhouse or garrison, its sentinel lampposts and tall palm trees bristling against the sky. A ragged wash of eucalyptus trees hangs over the freeway, their scaly limbs dwindle into a golf course swarming with tiny toiling figures pulling carts; and, although more eucalyptus hides the nearby sewage disposal plant, the unmistakable smell of harsh chemicals assails us. Dissonance bursts from the car radio; the air waves churn with conflict as two radio stations meet and war with each other. The sounds and the smells jar us, but we both anticipate clean calm air as soon as the freeway broadens, joins a second freeway and enters the country of the iron maidens.

The iron maidens are power installations that march beside us now, row upon row, each with three pairs of metal arms projecting stiffly from a central body pole, holding long dark loops of wire in their steel grasp. They stride and hum, hum and stride, leading us into a stony wilderness of quarries. The sign that dominates the rock quarries states tersely OWL ROCK COMPANY. Only the iron maidens can walk through these parts without falling down steep cliffs into funnels or machines that grind and spill out gray spume. Streams of gravel constantly descend toward some objective in the pits that lie below our line of vision. We glimpse gray-white rock piles and ash, a sudden open cleft that reveals water running past. The looming quarries subside, become a stretch of vegetation, a small truck farm where clumps of green plants grow, human figures bending over them.

The freeway leaps to the west, expands, presents us with a vista. It is like rushing into dawn after a squall at sea; we enter a valley placid and roseate, encircled by snow-tipped mountains. My daughter watches the ridges, the tiny white and pink houses, the pines and hair-line roads. "Mother," she warns, "don't miss the turn-off," but I have found the sign that spells out HOSPITAL and the small pointing arrow.

A town sits at the foot of the freeway. We pass a bus stop. A bench painted yellow and blue carries a six-pointed star and an advertisement for a mortuary upon its wooden back. Traffic lights blink and hold us motionless, release us to flow over the railroad tracks, to turn left and follow the green meadows and lawns of the City of Hope.

I drive cautiously. We have reached the city. We are both silent, brooding. What is she devising, does she loathe or does she draw strength from the carefully landscaped grounds, borders and gravelled paths that bend among roses and dahlia beds? Does she ever leave the environs of the city, when time passes too slowly there, and sit on these stone benches, or walk beneath the arbors; is she discovering the round mausoleums, the beehive tombs embellished with the words *in memory of*?

A driveway takes us to the rim of a stone fountain capped by a group of statuary that is meant to be a symbol of biological life and, therefore, literally, of hope. It is impossible not to stare at the group in the fountain, no matter how often I walk this way. Three figures dance above the gushing water: a man, a woman and a child, who is being passed from one pair of arms to another. They are stylized forms with perfectly blank faces, their arms curved boomerangs. My daughter turns her face to me which is mobile, alive and glowing. "Mother," she says, "I don't want to be here."

"Yes," I say. "I know."

The hospital building is a huge starfish, long arms radiating from a central corpus. It sucks us in, pulls us toward sea-green carpeted floors and aqua-tinted walls, cool corridors and the pulsations of laboratories and lounges. We are processed, brought to orange plastic cushions, left to wait. We are given over to time passing, passing, and to hope.

Hours later I leave. My daughter must stay at the hospital for a few days. She shrugs and relaxes. Her room is comfortable, there are flowers, the hummingbird feeder outside the window is stained a deep pink to attract the birds. She tells me what to bring when I visit her tomorrow: magazines, some apricots, a packet of yarn. I leave her in the many-celled city with its long arms, inside the starfish.

Outside it is dark night and the fountain lights are turned on. The stone statues glisten, fixed in their eternal dancing moment. I stop to look at them again and say: "Just so—man, woman, child..." The water surges and moves, I move on, continuing my return from Hope in darkness; but I understand every change, every phase of the journey. I drive through shadows past the cloud-covered mountains. Little can be seen now beyond the illuminated curves of the freeway, but I experience the reversals of returning in the fibers of my body.

I sense the presence of the truck farm when I pass it, as I do the quarries, the iron maidens, the sewage disposal plant, the golf course, the college, the cemetery. I perceive them all, touch them, taste them, feel them flow into my life. I know they are burning me, I know I shall see them forever.

Chapter 29

From Italy Paul's anxious voice surges over the telephone lines and shapes a series of questions.

"Oh, but it's too early to know if she'll respond," I explain, and, "Kellon won't make any predictions at this point. He's done another bone marrow—"

"What was that like?" Paul demands.

"Well, it was very cellular, like the last one. White cells are proliferating." Neither of us needs to be reminded what danger lies in this one symptom.

"How is she feeling, though?" he asks.

"A little bit uncomfortable." I decide not to mention the sores on her tongue or the facial swelling. "Once the new treatment takes hold, she'll be all right." I stand outside myself, appraising the confident tone of my voice.

He asks how the rest of us are faring and the line falls silent.

Before long Carol comes home to take up her textbooks and stitchery and let her infectious laughter ripple through the rooms and tug at the edges of my mind. Paul returns, too, shortly before her birthday. She is radiant, very nearly ecstatic, on the fifth of November. "I'm eighteen years old at last and people can finally start calling me an adult. Hooray!" she exults, tossing the words out over her shoulder while she ransacks the cupboards for vases to hold bunches of roses and chrysanthemums and powdery eucalyptus leaves. She will not allow Amy or Julie to help her, although one hand is preoccupied with an ice pack which she pats nervously against her face, still swollen and a bit lop-sided.

The radio begins to crackle with news bulletins about the results of the election that has just been concluded. Carol sighs. "If you'd only been a little more politically oriented, mom," she says, "and paid better attention to dates, I could've been born right before election day, instead of right after. That way, I could've voted this year."

Paul, being jocular: "Anyhow, Carol, you were born under the same sign I was—" He means the maternity ward, but Carol hastens to retort, "What sign exactly is that, daddy, the dollar sign?" and he shouts with laughter.

We sing happy birthday at the right moment: Paul, Amy and Julie carry the left-over cake and icecream out of the room. Facing Carol, a bit tongue-tied for some unaccountable reason and trying to overcome it, I repeat one more time, "Congratulations on being eighteen." My thoughts jostle against each other. Oh, how young she looks! collides with, but how mature she has gotten to be lately! and somewhere in between comes the warning, Watch out! She knows what you're thinking. She nearly always does these days....

"Stop worrying, mother," Carol says. "I'm going to live forever." She has intercepted my nascent thought.

I feel the pull of the invisible bond that links us. Ever since the beginning of relapse, earlier than that, I reflect, the bond has been tightening like a drawn cord until my awareness of her has become a kind of separate perception. When she is out of physical range sometimes I can sense exactly where she is or even hear the inflections of her speech, the laugh, the soft escaping sigh. On occasion I perceive her thoughts, as she so readily knows mine. When the linkage between us grows especially taut I imagine a beam of darkish light connecting me to her; it flares up and very fleetingly illuminates the uncharted course we follow together.

The earth revolves, the days become shorter, paler,

strung with mist and delicate gray rain. Treatment succeeds treatment. Carol endures more blood transfusions, further moments of rebellion and anger that subside into a numb resignation. "Mother, take me home from this place," she pleads. "Please, please, I feel like I'm dying here." It is a clear autumn day and the City of Hope glistens in the aftermath of a brief rainfall. She lifts her head; the pointed chin turns imperiously in my direction. "You think you can't do that. You think the City of Hope is going to save me." Helplessly I leave her late that same night, still pallid and beseeching, exhausted from tears and surrounded by a ring of rumpled paper tissues. The next day she greets me with a blunt pronouncement. "My doctor wants to do a bone marrow transplant. He just told me."

I am wordless, shocked.

"Mother, don't look like that. It's the very latest thing. Dr. Kellon says siblings—which would be Julie or Amy naturally—are the most qualified people, usually, as donors." Under her self-imposed calm a profound excitement is seething. She reaches out toward me impulsively.

"Oh, Carol," I cry. We are holding each other so close I can feel the intake of her breath and the pulsations of her heart. The blood transfusion just recently completed has left her cheeks rosy and brilliant. Gently I sprinkle the heated skin with water drops shaken from her drinking glass. I rock her in my arms as if I were carrying a small child, though, of course, she is now eighteen, a full-grown adult.

"Mother, I'm still your baby," she says perceptively, "and I'll always, always be..." Adult, adolescent, child, infant, she recedes within my arms and returns for a blinding scintilla of time to my womb.

Kellon talks cautiously to Paul and me about the proposed transplant. First of all, he says, it is a very recent method, only a year old. Not many transplants have actually been done. Secondly, the bone marrow used in the surgery must be completely compatible or the recipient's system will reject it. Thirdly, Amy and Julie, the most likely donors, must have their blood and lymphatic systems tested at the City of Hope, though the actual transplant, using the aspiration technique, would be performed at UCLA. "Think of it," the doctor concludes with emphasis, "as simply another form of therapy. As such, it may work—or it may not."

Chapter 30

As winter advances and the holidays arrive, my diary explodes into quick jottings and phrases. *Carol, nearly a week in Utah*, I scribble. *Back to final exams, Les, Debbie, Ron, Rick, Dennis, etc.* On the subject of the bone marrow transplant I wax more expressive.

Dr. Kellon acts jovial and is generous with information, if we could only understand it. He says both Amy and Julie are compatible blood types with Carol, but this is not enough, further "blood-tissue" tests must be run which he intends to supervise. He describes a mysterious concept called the HLA system that is concerned with matching immunities in the blood. "There's no immediate hurry," he says, ignoring any signs of strain on the part of his listeners. "All her counts appear to be on the upswing." Carol is wistful and excited simultaneously, Paul moody, Julie and Amy highly-strung, each smouldering with the desire to be donor.

The suspense hangs on. Carol confides in Gayle who also has two siblings and might herself be a candidate for a transplant. Gayle shows a lively interest. "I think it would be great," she says. "I heard about a girl who had one done last month and so far it's been practically perfect."

Carol picks up some of Gayle's enthusiasm. "Think about this, mother," she says. "What if the two of us, Gayle and me, had the surgery done together, on some date after the New Year? Both of us could be at UCLA, roommates or something!"

Much, much later Kellon admits to me in confidence that Gayle's blood is simply too unstable even for typing at this time.

Mid-December. Five Azacytidine treatments, four units of blood. A few pinkish boils stir beneath the surface of Carol's skin. She covers them up and begins making Christmas decorations, a wreath out of bay leaves, berries and cinnamon sticks and a red and white angel constructed over a plastic cone, dressed in ribbons and white lace.

Christmas Day. We exchange gifts under the steady regard of the red and white angel. I activate the tape that is to run all day and record our conversations in front of the hearth and on the deck of the *Chipsee*. *High spirits,* I write hurriedly that evening. *Carol's counts still rising and the number of blast cells much reduced.*

Dr. Kellon phones in the results of the blood tissue tests the day after Christmas. I underline the date with great bitterness: December 26, 1974. No go, no match, no donor.

A despondent Carol sits at the desk swinging her foot. "Well, am I going to die? Shall I ask Kellon?" Her father calls from Chicago and simply refuses to believe the message she gives him. "This is one of Carol's 'kidders,' isn't it?" he asks me. "She doesn't mean that about the test results, does she?"

"It's true," I reply sadly. "But she's trying not to think about it. She's moving." I watch her carry the orange fern stand out of the room. After a week of considerable argument Paul and I have both capitulated to her desire to move into a large apartment with her friends, Les and Debbie. She is moving out, piece by piece. The bedside table, the radio and the clock have already departed, I realize, putting down the telephone. Looking distressed and pensive, Carol studies the remaining furniture along the wall. I understand: she wants to move, but she also wants to stay here.

I lose myself in the back yard, avoiding the packing up procedure and conscious of a dull pain that must be eased.

She packs and then goes out with her friend Fred to attend a young people's meeting; I glimpse her stretched across the water bed, reading the Bible, when I retire and the long day finally dissolves.

January. I am writing less, reading more—the Irish mystic AE, Gertrude Stein, Plutarch, Edith Hamilton's *Mythology*. Hamilton, the classicist who was made an honorary citizen of Athens. I jot down my dreams, make staccato notations in the diary. In spite of the doctor's warnings I feel the need for rhythm and movement so strongly that I take up swimming again with an inner surge of relief, almost of benediction.

Much support from the Monday night prayer group. No word from the Charismatics. Night and day I repeatedly urge my mind to project images of the well Carol, wholeness and healing, but these interior visions are at sharp variance with the physical reality I encounter whenever I meet my daughter. I cannot will away her tiredness or the re-emerging red dots, the bruises, the small inflammations.

We meet frequently; the apartment lies only a few miles distant from the house. Though she is as affectionate as ever, I perceive it is her intention to rely on me less and sense that she is caught in a sort of alternating current, back-to-me, away-from-me. "This is my illness, I can deal with it," she says driving herself to the City of Hope without me. But she finds a reason to stop by the house afterwards and engage in a long conversation. "Kellon can always tell when I need a transfusion by looking at my mouth...and when the new blood comes in, why I feel it....I feel so very warm all over."

We make elaborate arrangements for me to visit her at the apartment, once she and the two roommates are completely settled. Still, somehow, in spite of the planning, the directions are inadequate or I misinterpret them, and I wait at the wrong place in an empty parking lot. She is not there, I cannot find her. I pace the asphalt. My vocal chords vibrate with low mourning sounds, almost a keening, quite beyond my control. Some desolate ruin within me speaks. What is wrong? Can she be playing a trick on me, would she?

Carol darts around a corner, effusive and apologetic. I don't hear her explanations. My relief is so great I clutch both of her hands. She is real, after all, then. The sense of loss I felt in the empty parking lot is the illusion.

Heightened emotions attend my whole visit and I retain only a few quick bright impressions like daubs of color on a painter's palette. The living room, cool and dim, green ferns, philodendron. Carol's room, long, yellow and green, the two zebra finches chirping wildly. Posters, ceramics, a seed box, spice cabinet in the kitchen. Cheerful, lively. People in and out. "Do you like it, mom?" she asks and then, hesitantly, "Do you miss me?"

Two days pass before she stops by to borrow the electric mixer. Wearing a dazed expression, she wanders about, lightly touching a vase or a lamp, petting Blackie and the new striped tabby, Kitten. She tells me in an off-hand manner that Dr. Kellon is out of town. "Will you go with me to the hospital for treatment today, mother?"

Dr. Fayhe is substituting for Dr. Kellon. He spends a lot of time looking at Carol's latest counts, calls me in, clears his throat, and then speaks the words I least expected to hear. "Your daughter is holding her own, Mrs. Trautmann." He repeats the statement, that bleak and wholly meaningless pronouncement of the summer before last, uttered so often when Carol's life teetered in the balance. He has something else to add. "Dr. Kellon may decide to change her course of treatment soon."

Enveloped in a trance and unseeing, I walk back to the car. My uneven course accidentally cuts across Carol's path. She is cradling her left elbow in her right hand, and cries out: "Mother, watch it! You're going to run me down!" I execute a complicated physical maneuver to avoid a collision, feeling, as I do so, the abrupt slide into the cold gravel pit again, the invisible water rising past my nostrils and eye sockets, change of color, change of temperature, an iciness that ripples clear to the earth's core, the urgency of my groping.

We stop at home. Carol is contrite. She wants to make me a nightgown in preparation for the vascular surgery I have scheduled in February, saying "It's your turn to enter the hospital. I'll be visiting you for a change!"

I decline the offer, but she is determined to make me something, a long skirt, she decides, and shows me a swatch of crinkly sprigged plisse in fresh spring colors. "Like it?"

"Yes, very much, well, all right, then, thanks." My tongue thickens and stumbles as I watch her depart and the house turns labyrinthine, filled with underwater passages that lengthen and darken in front of me.

In her chapter about the Trojan war Edith Hamilton takes up the story of Aeneas, Trojan survivor. Hamilton's words cause echoes of Latin to stir in my head, reviving long-forgotten phrases and imagery. Memories of the Sybil are renewed, wise-woman and seer, the guide who enables Aeneas to find the golden bough. I read again how essential this branch is for the safety of the traveller who, like the Trojan, attempts to reach the country of the dead. Carrying the golden bough in one hand, the Sybil leads the adventurer to the entrance of the afterworld, which lies above steaming Lake Avernus and is not as difficult to find as most people think, she says, since 'all night long, all day, the doors to dark Hades lie open...'

I bring the *Mythology* and my diary with me when I enter the community hospital for surgery.

CAROL WRITING

Carol writes as if a brisk off-shore wind were at her back propelling her through life. Urgency animates the irregular script and hasty spelling of the papers she accumulates at every level of the public school system, kindergarten to community college; but it is particularly pronounced in the spontaneous writing that takes so many different forms—marginalia, comments scribbled wherever her fancy directs, notes addressed to herself or to close friends, isolated philosophical paragraphs in the middle of lecture notes, a prose poem, a short story. A collector of memorabilia of all sorts, she collects words as well, compiling long lists, a few of them meant for the classroom, others justified by the intrinsic pleasure they give her.

The first list shows up in a stock market game she plays with her sisters when she is seven years old and uses a clipboard and pencil and squares of paper to invent imaginary companies and shares in coal, corn, cotton, iron, lumber, fish, fur. The first poems appear at almost the same time.

> birds are little things
> you feel like hugging them and thanking God for
>   making them
> they sing to you in the morning
> Oh, they sing so sweet

> trees are very wonderful
> they are company to you when you are alone
> they are very good friends
> they almost talk to you
> when the wind goes through their leaves you can
> tell them secrets and problems that you have
> and yet they won't tell anyone

> When I feel lonely and left out
> I go outside
> I climb a tree
> I think to me

> what would it be to live alone?
> to live alone, to live alone
> with no one else, no, no one else
> what would it be to live alone?

What Happened to Little Carol is an unfinished short story that occupies several pages in a spiral notebook.

> Once there was a little girl. Her name was little Carol Jordan. Carol was always getting into other people's things. She got into everything and anything. One day when her mother had to go to a very important person's house, Carol went along and got into the bathroom and looked at all the cupboards and drawers and found brushes, curlers, soap, combs, cold cream, bubble bath, bobby pins, scrub brush, hair spray, hand lotion, toothpaste, shampoo, powder, pins, band aids, first aid kit... they went to a department store and Carol went to a cashier and snooped in all the money, then the department store lady yelled at her and told her mother.... They went to another store and Carol wanted to know if the dog food tasted good, so she opened a pack and tasted it. 'How can dogs stand that stuff?' Carol said. When they got to the pet store she opened all the birds' cages and the other cages too and every dog and cat was running around and all the birds were flying loose....

While still in grade school she signs an irate memorandum to herself with the words *from the future Dr. Trautmann*, commenting crookedly across blue paper that,

> lots of children do not like school, but it helps us learn. If you grow up and become a doctor you will have to know arithmetic. If you become a writer you will have to know how to write and if you become a nurse you will have to spell long hard words....

When she receives an A-plus on her state of Wisconsin report she congratulates herself by writing:

> Carol, this is a very good report and I know it took a lot of time and effort. But you must remember your margins! But only 4 miss speiled words is very good!

In 1965 she is nine years old. She draws up a list of her favorite activities: watch birds, collect rocks and shells, watch the stars, study leaves, look at trees, swim, play with pets, take guitar lessons. She says farewell to grade school and the first decade of her life in a page of book reviews written for the school magazine, praising several adventure stories fulsomely and one book in particular because it is "full of hilarious stories about noodle heads all over the world."

In junior high school Carol aligns herself with a secret club, the Faithful Four, whose structure necessitates a mass of papers, a mysterious code, a format of questions and answers, a list of "appropriate things to say at meetings" and a few original rules:

> Do not take money from our bank or you will have to pay twice as much as you took.... If only one person is coming to the meeting, call it all off.... If any one breaks a rule of the club, she will have to drink salt, sugar and pepper in a teaspoon of water.

Carol writes:

> I always have a lot of thoughts, but one of my main thoughts is how I can stay out of trouble at home and school. I don't want to get in trouble at home because I hate to have my parents mad at me and I don't want to get grounded.

Among a group of short stories appears an adventure tale about her first space voyage to the land of the Woodlings, peculiar robots fashioned entirely out of wood who scold Carol with the flashing electronic sentences that crackle across their foreheads:

We know why you are here and it is a pretty dumb reason. We know all there is to know, so don't think you're so smart. Now you can say whatever you want to, but no wise-cracks!

The Chief Woodling is an intolerant type who cannot endure any interruptions while he watches television. Carol laughs at the wrong time and the Woodling blows up her space ship.

In a poetry notebook Carol asks:

> I do not know what I shall be
> if I should teach or type or try for politics
> it worries me
> but is it any wonder why?
> the future comes so fast
> as the time flies by

When she is thirteen years old she is assigned to write an essay on courage:

> I think the best meaning I could put together for this word would be the ability to act effectively in the face of danger or difficulty. That is, the ability to look straight at danger or hardship and not be turned aside from doing what I really want to do and think I should do…You can't be afraid of the world or run away from things that you dislike. Courage is a necessity of life. You must have it.

The note writing, the lists and the comments along the margins of papers proliferate as she makes her way through high school. She is too busy to keep a conventional diary, but the notes written to herself and to her sisters, parents and friends serve very nearly the same purpose. Once in a while the notes extend themselves and become a chronicle. Three pages of sprawling extravagant handwriting record a short romance that occupied her thoughts briefly during her freshman year:

> Monday, December 7—A wonderful day! R. might like me!

Friday, Dec. 11—Today was the best day of my entire life, the day of all the hopes, dreams and wishes that I have had for 3 months. Yet I barely even talked to R. He told Debbie that he *did* like me!

Tuesday, Dec. 15—Almost as terrible as yesterday. Didn't say a word to R. I sat with Les at lunch in front of the auditorium steps and cussed R. and the world out even though he didn't hear me.

Dec. 16—It rained a lot at lunch. We were standing about 4 feet away from each other, but our backs were turned. I was in a good, but weird mood. Not much happened with him. Maybe tomorrow will be a better day. It's back to looking and not talking.

Dec. 17—I give up! There are other chickens in the coop! I'm going to face up to facts and try to forget R. Tomorrow I'll feel better...

Carol writes:

My main problem with the English language is spelling and neatness—still.

As of November 18, 1971, Carol owns the green sweater which Amy still has the right to wear when she wants, maximum use for Amy four times a month.

> I have a lot to tell you about last night and I don't even know why I'm writing this note since I see you next period....So, with all my confusion inside of me bottled up, I stand alone feeling like the whole world is against me, not knowing what to do. And you have been getting mad at me the past few days, I really don't mean to start fights, but you seem bellicose to me. I'm kind of afraid that our friendship isn't as strong as it used to be, but I hope it is because it is one of the only things that means a lot to me and that I treasure....
>
> Well, when I went to the library, I was walking up the walk to the door and everything seemed normal. All of a sudden I heard the sound of breaking glass,

> I looked around and saw the glass door of the library shatter. I was very shocked and just stood there amazed. People started to point at the shattered door and stared. No one was able to figure out what had happened... Later, the police came...

> Today is Julie's birthday, happy birthday
> Julie, you better fix my mobile or else
> I have a stomach ache
> I wonder when Debbie is coming over
> I wonder when the women in the living room are
>   going to leave
> I have to learn my French conversation
> finish my map
> study my triangles for geometry
> and read my book if I want to but I don't want to
>   I'm bored, bored, bored

The list of favorite activities compiled during her sophomore year is not too different from the inventory taken seven years earlier; climbing trees, swimming, being with animals and flowers still rate very high, but she has added driving a car, parties and rap sessions. "I like to do things that I enjoy with people that I like and things that don't cost much money."

The myth that she composes for English class is entitled *How the Giraffe Got his Long Neck*.

> Once long ago in the deepest jungles of Africa there was a goddess. She was the goddess of the creatures and plants in the jungle and the plains of all Africa. She lived among the animals, trees, the strange and beautiful flowers that she had created. Her name was Kyteekee, meaning 'all powerful.' Now Kyteekee loved all her animals dearly, but she had been getting a little upset with one small animal lately. He was called a deeraffe. This creature was very small and delicate like a tiny deer of today.

Carol's myth states that the perfection and delicacy of the

deeraffe cause him to make fun of other animals and eventually even the goddess, herself. Kyteekee, who slips and falls in the mud, is made angry by the deeraffe's mockery. She grabs him by the neck and tugs away, saying:

> 'Because you are always jeering at everyone, I'm going to change you into the strangest looking animal of earth, so that all who meet you will laugh at you.' And Kyteekee named her new creation a jeer-affe, to remind him always why he had been punished.... Even today if you ever travel to Africa you will see the jeer-affe, whose name is now spelled giraffe, running around the plains trying to hide his long neck.

She critiques John Gunther's volume, *Death, Be Not Proud.*

> John Gunther's son had character. He was sick and could hardly move his hands... but he did almost impossible feats in this condition because he had the will.... In the short time that John had left, he did what he was good at doing and by really trying he was able to finish school. He was probably sad that he wasn't able to live longer and that no one had invented some cure for him, because if he had lived he might have done a lot of good for the world.

In 1972 she jots down more columns of words in her notebooks, lists of medical terms, political phrases and topics, recipes, words that she likes. She writes an imaginary letter from parents living on the eastern sea-coast to a son in the wild west of the 1890's.

> Your mom is wondering when you plan to settle down. She says that the women out west aren't fit for you, that a son needs a real fine woman who'll make a wife and mother, not the strong, rugged, fearless ones that go riding around shooting people like Calamity Jane or those saloon girls that will never conform to anything.

A prose-poem separates itself from the notes and recipes.

If you have ever walked through a field of daisies
blowing with the wind
you understand beauty
these flowers seem to whisper to you
they bring happiness and put joy in your heart
daisies are happiness and beauty

At the community college the wind that is blowing at her back hurtling her through life increases in volume and the hurried, self-scrutinizing comments appear less often, yet they can still be found, wandering in and out among the pages of her lecture notes.

I feel my mind is really working and wondering and I am questioning everything that anyone says. I am learning how to be more aware.

To really communicate one person must understand the other's position and point of view. The main problem is trying to express a clear picture for someone else to imagine....like, for instance, with mom and my moving out of the house...at first, she just couldn't understand...

If you are happy, so are others, and isn't this what God promises all along, happiness, eternal life?

Mom wanted to quit being a girl scout leader and the person that was going to take her place had four kids and got pregnant again, so she wouldn't have any time to take the training...I said 'Yes, she will be able to do it. Something is going to happen. She won't have this fifth baby.' Two weeks later the woman was in the hospital with a miscarriage. Don't know why I said what I did. How did I know?

Her familiar ever-recurring lists appear on lined paper deep within the notebooks or scattered freely among reminders of visits to the hospital, warnings about tests, predictions of final grades. One of the last lists catalogues the things that were on her mind just before Easter week, 1975: laundry, phone mom, term paper, bank, make plaque for daddy, river trip.

The allure of words still holds and endures as long as breath itself. Back in third grade the small dictionary she compiled when her hand was still struggling to bring the unwieldy letters down to tolerable size ends with two words—Wisconsin and yesterday. The last word list in her college notebook ends pin-pointed on a dazzle of light. *Lucidity, rebirth,* Carol writes.

Chapter 31

At the hospital my horizon is limited to a square of window revealing an overcast sky and to a length of corridor in front of the elevators which I traverse the day after surgery, learning to walk again. I stagger back and forth on this narrow runway, physically unsure, emotionally spent.

Paul and my daughters bring me presents. Carol ties a ribbon in my hair and gives me a book of prose poems illustrated with delicate crayon drawings and entitled *The Colors of Time*. February is a *period of meditation*, the book says, *when days curl closer to each other seeking shelter from the cold and the darkness.* Its colors, I notice, turning the pages, are brown and purple, charcoal and winter white.

The charcoal and white colors of February extend from the hospital room to the home I return to where my family moves under restraint, lacking their usual spontaneity, and plants, animals and birds wait with a hushed gray expectancy.

Valentine's Day. Carol comes home late in the afternoon to get ready for a party at the apartment; she likes to dress here, she says, and she wants to show me her new gown. Her eyes look feverish. Her temperature is 101 and rising, so I notify Dr. Kellon who obligingly phones in a prescription for an antibiotic. I do not even suggest that she go to the City of Hope.

She puts on the soft new dress, long-skirted and sprinkled with sprightly orange and blue designs, and meets me in the kitchen. For some reason the ceiling light is turned off and we stand in front of the stove while an illuminated gas ring forms a circlet of blue flame. She lights a cigarette, bending down to the circle of fire, her profile a single shining unbroken line in the dusky room.

It is impossible to say where the moment takes us. The kitchen walls dull to clay. The profile suspended above the blue flames has bronzed, the features enamelled into a look that is Egyptian and archaic. The slender neck elongates, the hair darkens; above the high forehead a conical headdress sweeps bordered by a stripe of gold. Helplessly I name her Nefertiti scarcely breathing the syllables into a stillness that deepens and spreads. I am becalmed, mute. She stirs at last. "What did you say, mother?"

"You remind me of somebody. Shall I tell you about her?"

She listens, the sculptured and masked planes of her face rigid, the immobile gaze held transfixed by the fire. In an agony of compulsion and fear I grope for the light switch. My daughter is restored to pallor and movement.

She visits the house often during these days, evidently caught in a tug-of-war with nostalgia and swept by the alternating current of away-from-me, back-to-me. She cultivates a new formality. "Are you certain it's all right if I borrow the iron?" she asks politely. Eagerly I await the winged smile and the clear chiming laughter.

One Saturday morning I unexpectedly find her bent over the card catalogue at the public library. She sits engrossed, fingers among the cards. The spontaneous greeting on my lips subsides because conditions are altering too rapidly for speech. The moment transforms. The library dims. What I assume are tall bookcases become the shadowy boles of trees. Carol's pale arms are traced with a slight transparent layer of bark, the finger nails attenuate into narrow dendritic shapes, her hair reveals leafy patterns through which the pink and white of her blouse shimmers and blossoms. So once the nymph pursued by the sun god became other substance, flesh into wood, blood into the sweet rushing fluids of the tree. The gaze that languidly shifts and focuses upon me beams out of a different epoch, from forests and rivers of antiquity filtered through the streaming millennia.

Time shivers. "Mother, hello!" She reclaims the present. The encompassing forest becomes a library, the trees revert to shelves and stacks, the pink and white bloom re-structures itself into the blouse she is wearing.

"You haven't called me up for ages," she says accusingly.

My reply is close to a stammer. "But, Carol, I'm never sure exactly when....whether I should phone or not." Her new freedom, I do not wish to diminish that.

"You can phone me any time, mother. Please call up and talk to me any time you want!"

I consider her new life style which includes a good many elements of the old: the friendships, parties, exams, a social calendar framed by the iron claims of treatment and granting little space to leisure and reflection. She is reaching out to me just the same. Some portion of her loneliness is communicating with my own.

"Carol, I miss you," I say. "I miss having you at the house."

"Yes, I know," she answers. "But don't worry, mother, I'll be back."

End of the month, another trip to Duarte with Carol that concludes late in the day. I wave farewell, speeding her on to the apartment and step back into a silent realm where a chastened watchdog guides me past empty rooms. The house seems hollow. I go down a maze of plastered walls whose rough textures feel unfamiliar as I graze them with my hands. Under the contact separate atoms of wood and paint and plaster leap and tremble. A dimly echoing laundry room. The harsh sound of the back door slamming shut.

I am looking at the landscape of my own backyard through a finely adjusted lens; what I see lies over the familiar as if a water-color sketch had been hastily brushed on and left to streak and mingle with the original background. The lens re-focuses. Nothing looks as it did when I last viewed the yard in the early morning. The soil which lay at the foot of the hill, freshly turned, in preparation for a garden, has vanished or has been painted over. Instead of earth, lake water steams, the surface of a cauldron, Lake Avernus, if I were to put a name to it, emitting vapor, thin shreds that drift, nebulous and without form until they reach the banks and then take on a gray and more substantial outline, assume features, garments and emblems, becoming images with every appearance of shadowy life. As images or apparitions they take their place in a solemn procession that winds up the hillside.

Even the trees of the landscape are askew, distorted by the lens that pulls at my eyes. The orange and avocado trees have stiffened into austere uncompromising lines. They lean inwardly, their branches frame a yawning cavern that gapes wide at the exact point where the path ends. The gates of the afterworld are standing open, as the Roman writer insists they always do, and through the dark entrance I see the Eumenides pass, their heavy robes swirling; a formal cordon of hamadryads; the three Moirae lifting up the distaff and shears for dispensing the thread of human life; a chain of mountain oreads; the proud winged Nemesis; Nox and Hemera, night and day, who lead the dawn Eos, blinded by the light from her own forehead; the grieving Niobe; Arachne, Eurydice, the stern incorruptible Styx and many others I cannot recognize or have never known about.

The last figures to arise out of the cloudy lake place a glittering gold branch at the foot of the hill. As the lens drops away and my vision steadies, I call out to the vanishing images: "Don't go! Don't leave yet, please!" They have already gone. Frustration fills me to overflowing. "Keep the golden bough!" I storm after them. "Why bring me gifts? Just answer—Can you help my daughter? Can you give her life?" The evening wind, beginning to rustle the edges of the ivy, catches my words and carries them back to me. The branch which I bend over and pick up from the ground does not bear a vestige of gold, but shines with the glossy greenness of the avocado boughs soughing over my head.

The branches are weeping together and as I listen it seems

to me that the earth spirit weeps with them, a lament for the many shapes of death that daily, hourly, are laid within innumerable passages. The dirge rises from battlefields and burial shafts, the corpses of men and wolves, the insensate wings of the mayfly, the drying petals of the flower that blooms one solitary day and is gone, the pyres and tombs, wherever death walks and that is everywhere. Sinking into the freshly dug soil underneath me, I feel the clods fashioned from death, animal flesh, decayed plants, the bones of women, mouldering trees, skeletons of insects and rodents. Earth soil, death-made, mocks me. Life is doom and death and I weep, too, as the earth does, for the procession of death, the silent unspeaking dead.

Shadows form and elongate. Some presence towers above me in the half-light. Who would keep this mournful vigil with me? I wonder and look up. Never before have I seen the Companion as she now presents herself—in an aspect of immensity that dwarfs the trees, magnifies her limbs and the features of her face and gives her the burning compassionate glance of an immortal. She carries a long unlighted torch.

I gather the hem of her massive cape and bury my face in its folds, believing that I should control my tears. She tells me to weep. Her large smooth hand caresses my shoulders in the gesture of a consoling mother. The light strong voice utters words that ripple and enfold me very much as her cape does. "I am always near. You are never alone, for I am as close as your own breath. Whenever you look for me, I approach."

She stands beside me tall and luminous and gentle. The torch in her hand is alight with fire. She tosses it heavenward and the flaming brand sails across the night sky ushering in the stars.

March. Carol comes home in the afternoon to rest on the water-bed and play with Blackie. She brings a book with her, *Stay of Execution* by Stewart Alsop, which is the author's commentary upon his own on-going experiences with leukemia. He writes about the inevitability of confronting death, "that good old white-haired uncle," his favorite symbol. Carol plans to review the book for her health class.

"Please don't read this one," I say. "Change the topic, choose something else." She shrugs. At the last moment she ignores the book and leaves it on the couch.

Her gums are bleeding. "Well, I can't do much about them," she says. "I'll just get some mouthwash at the drugstore." We look closely at each other. A faint half-smile brushes her mouth, but the eyes are unsmiling. We embrace.

"You are just exactly beautiful," I tell her, "and I love you very much."

She loves me, too, she says gravely.

Chapter 32

For the first time within my memory Carol insists that she wants to go to the City of Hope. Her gums are swollen, temperature close to 102, an infection almost certainly present. Blood stains on her striped pillow at the apartment.

"Mother, am I real sick?" she questions over and over.

"Dear, please don't worry. It will be all right." I drive past the slate-colored mountains which are barely visible through their aura of mist.

"But am I really sick?" Carol persists. "Will they treat the infection intravenously?"

Hours afterward, stepping out of the back entrance to Wing Five, I carry away with me a mental photograph as fresh as any brand-new print. Carol, wearing a pink dotted swiss robe, Steve on one side of her, Rick on the other, balanced for all the world like a pair of courtiers; the green stuffed frog and the brown kaola bear alternating as supports and steadying Carol's forearm during injections, their fur bulging and spattered a bit; the asymmetrical positions of a candy box and a vase of flowers. My eye retains the exact angle taken by a curve of plastic tubing, the small pyramid made by toes pointed together under the bedsheet, the orange accent of pimento in a jar of olives. The photograph begins to complicate, each detail elaborating with the feather-like delicacy of a Seventeenth Century flower painting.

Carol's telephone call startles me early the next morning.

She is in profound distress, her voice scarcely audible. Her friend Gayle died in February, two weeks ago. Dr. Kellon has just told her. Died of bleeding in the brain, the onrush of too many white cells, Carol laments brokenly. She cries, I cry, hard driving tears.

I find some words. "But no one ever really dies. They just change, take on a different form." She welcomes my words, whispers that Dr. Kellon will be starting a new treatment tonight. However, when I reach the hospital, the nurse is already in the room adjusting the paraphernalia to begin a series of cytoxin and cytosine injections, or the C. and C., as she calls this treatment, which is to be administered around the clock at ten and two and six. Carol, having misunderstood her doctor's directive, is washing her hair in the shower. She emerges explosively.

"I want to wash it while I can," she shouts through the dribbles of water. "It's going to fall out, you know!" She blows her nose fiercely and demands that the injection be postponed. Disconcerted, the nurse leaves.

I sit in silence while my daughter weeps for Gayle and for her own yellow hair soon to be sacrificed. Resentfully she turns the hair dryer up to high heat. The dryer whistles as it blows, repeating a thin slurring note. Now, now, the dryer whirs, spinning out a skein of words. Love, how we learn what it is, now! This is my beloved, my beloved daughter; live then this very present moment, live the instant fully. Aware, be aware of the instant, enter it, every facet, the pain, the rage, the accusing eyes. Be the anger, the pain, the shrill whistle of the dryer, the muttering of the television set in the corner, the luster of red-gold flowers, the light in this room, now.

The nurse Kathy motions me into the hall. "I've seen good results from this treatment," she says. "As for the side effects, I've been advising Carol that not everyone loses hair with the C. and C. Some do, some don't. It's not certain."

"Carol is terribly upset just now," I venture.

"Oh, of course. We all understand. She *should* feel anger. She *should* cry. She's a young girl and she's doing badly and wistfully, the absent friend, the contestant who has just abandoned the race.

The director of Social Services does not hesitate to speak of Gayle and people's attitudes toward death. "No one, however old," he tells me, "is ever resigned to illness and death. Age has nothing to do with it. Death grows no easier. One does not become seasoned to the idea... Courage is important, very crucial." He pays me a kind of tribute. "You will be strong," he says, "whenever strength is needed."

The air throngs with death. The actress Susan Hayward dies. Aristotle Onassis dies. The Brazilian father who was flown to the City of Hope from Rio de Janeiro last month dies. The widow, ringed by her family in the T.V. lounge, gesticulates, all black eyes and nervous motion. The young son, she vows, is now to become the head of the family. A daughter tells me that her mother has had no practical experience of any kind; she has never computed a bank balance or signed a check. The family business, financial obligations, in short, everything, falls on the shoulders of the brooding young man who frowns and stares at his mother.

Over television, the life cycle of bees. A camera unrelentingly examines the moment of death for worker bees, the death of the queen. We are a civilization obsessed by death, preoccupied with ignoring it.

Carol talks to me about death. "Gayle was the only person I could really confide in around here. She was so nice. Everyone loved her. She was always so funny! And I'm the irritating one!" Her brusque gesture checks me. "Do you think Gayle is alive now, mother?" The sharp gaze, the hurt, must be met and answered.

"Yes."

"How do you know?"

I understand what she is asking—the question that underlies every other question, old as humanity, that smiles out at us obliquely from all the death masks—what is reality? There are many answers. I know that my father's books contain his own individual answer; that every religion replies to this question; science, skepticism, logic, the world, all have their statements ready.

I draw a long breath. "Inner experience tells me, Carol, my own life tells me what I need to know about death."

She nods gently.

"Many years ago, before you were born, somebody I loved very much died—and it was different, a drowning, but I was nowhere near when it took place and I knew nothing at all about the circumstances."

She waits.

"Well, you see, my friend came back to me. Immediately, right after it happened. As a living presence, invisible except for a kind of radiance; and I felt the presence, we communicated with each other...and so, love and on-going life, you see, do break through barriers—silence, invisibility, even."

She is relaxed, head tilted back upon the pillow. "But why are we afraid to die?"

"The unknown frightens us."

"Do you think Gayle suffered when she died?"

"No, I do not."

She sighs. "Mother, I know Gayle is alive somewhere, too." She straightens up slowly. "Please, though, tell me what you intend to write to her mother. And then I'd like to take a walk upstairs through the children's ward."

We find the door that leads to the top floors. The stairs wind steeply past walls painted with bright cartoon murals. Babies, their heads close-shaven, regard us stoically from their cribs. Other children wave as we go by on our journey to the playground at the roof top where colored blocks, cloth dolls, story books and beads are heaped in orderly piles. We stand beside a railing above the familiar vista of rose gardens and sleek lawns.

"Kim was treated here." Carol looks about her. "And I could've been treated in this ward, too. With everyone who plays on this roof. I counted fifteen children as we went by." She sits on the parapet and says not a word more until we arrive at her room again and the white bedsheet is pulled up to her throat. She takes my hand. "Listen, I've been keeping a secret from you, but I really want you to know about it. So I'm going to tell you now." She watches my face. "Well, the other day—well, Ron, you know him now and daddy does too—anyhow, he took me to an old building somewhere in downtown Los Angeles." Her eyes widen. I can see the iris change color. "Honest, mom, I don't know exactly where we were—a church or a shrine of some sort, though, some place where a real old man blessed me. Mom, he could have been a hundred years old, he was older than grandma."

"Yes."

"He told the people there all about me and they crowded around and said they would pray for me. And then he blessed me again and there was a statue of the madonna in the room and—" She closes her eyes. "I felt different afterwards. I can't really describe it. But I said I would go back there again." A long period of silence envelops us. "Ron believes that I'm going to get well. But, mother, if it happens—Well, you have to consider it, everyone thinks about death, you know. If it happens, I'm not afraid."

She throws her arms around my neck. "Mother, I love you so much." She cleaves to me, tells me what lies close to her heart. When, eventually, I am obliged to leave the hospital, I resonate with her voice and the words and phrases I cannot even recall later on, so heady and empowering are the emotions that pervade me. The high commitment to joy she makes pours through my being also, like a limpid stream in summer.

St. Patrick's Day. Carol's breakfast tray disports a slice of green and white frosted cake and a tiny Erin Go Braugh flag stuck in a pot of flourishing shamrocks. A holiday mood invades Wing Five.

There is no talk of death today. Dr. Kellon, Carol says, is searching for a bone marrow donor; a transplant is still a possibility. Her platelet count is up, the hemoglobin at the twelve mark. She's having lots of visitors. Her face beams when I repeat word for word her father's long distance telephone message from Italy.

During some slack time after lunch I ramble through the extensive grounds that surround the City of Hope, losing my way more than once among the terraces and buildings.

Repeatedly, it seems almost by pre-arrangement, I end up scrutinizing the façade of the weathered structure known as Hillquit where tuberculosis patients were formerly housed during the early days of the medical research center.

Hillquit is flanked by a row of large tattered eucalyptus trees. It is only when I examine them closely, walking near to the dusty branches and peering past the flaking bark at the gray trunks that I see certain of these trees wear metal plaques. The plaques are chained about the tree trunks like necklaces or charm bracelets and are engraved with names and dates. They are, in fact, memorials.

The wind has blown a considerable scattering of leaves, bark slivers and pods upon the grass. The impression of their fragrance and shivering silver-green movement goes with me when I re-enter the corridors of Wing Five and almost without reflecting upon the matter, I describe the trees to Carol. Her response is instantaneous. "Oh, mother, can I have a tree, promise me, can I?"

I am unprepared for this reaction and my face shows it.

She repeats her request. "Promise me, mother, promise me, please."

I promise her a tree.

At home Carol's mood reverses. She phones the apartment and learns that her finches are "puffed up" and listless. She postulates an infection and frantically consults the veterinarian for advice. The glass bubble planter she recently filled with ivy and fern is badly chipped. One of her philodendron wilts on the hearth. For these and other offenses we are all roundly accused of neglect and then fully exonerated, as she hugs us and apologizes for "being so irritating." She is weary of the hospital, she explains, so exasperated she left early, before any of the laboratory results had been determined.

A few days later Carol bursts into the house, ecstatic, glowing. She is on her way back from the hospital. "Mother, oh mother!" she sings out. "Guess what the lab tests show, guess! *No* blast cells anywhere, good platelet count, everything normal, the way it should be!" She dances me through the kitchen. "I've been crying all the way home, I'm so happy!" She cries and laughs, can hardly find breath enough to describe her doctor's reactions. Usually, she says, such a lab report means that the patient will go into remission. "Dr. Kellon wants to repeat this same treatment in just one week; he's going to keep after it!" We are both weeping and laughing. She calls her father at his office and phones Les and Debbie, too, as soon as she can. "Les, the morning I left the City of Hope, you remember, the new treatment, the hurry I was in and everything—well, that morning my blood was perfectly normal. It was just like yours!"

The first day of Easter vacation. Exuberant, encouraged by her doctor's words and the laboratory testing, Carol plans to enjoy the next five days before treatment is resumed. She is going on another camping trip to the Colorado river with her friends. Sleeping bags are stashed quickly in the back seat of the Monte Carlo next to the blue suitcase and other camp gear.

The advance guard of vacationing teen-agers is already down at the river. Last minute delays, a few changes in the arrangements: Carol and Les and Christy will leave together and make a fast detour east of Whittier to pick up another friend, Terry. And so the Monte Carlo pulls slowly down the driveway in the early morning darkness, Carol next to its driver, talking rapidly, her eyes scanning the sky for some hint of dawn. The next stop will be Terry's house.

The March winds have been mustering throughout the day. Small craft warnings are posted along the coasts. Paul and I, sleeping fitfully, can hear the humming of the power lines that lead from the house to the garage into the shop. The weather stripping around the front door shrills, twigs drag across the roof.

"Are these the Santa Ana winds?" I ask Paul. "I thought they only blew in summer."

"Oh, I think they can blow any time," he says. "But this wind isn't coming from the desert."

Spring storm. So I identify the sounds before falling asleep and they mingle in dreams with the March winds of my childhood, the blasts that could send ripples of late powdery snow to cover the earth even in spring, winds with no hint of moderation to them, only a raw ferocity and turbulence.

Chapter 33

A tree falls somewhere in the night. Succumbing to the frenzy of the spring winds, its trunk cracks and splits, the flailing arms go down; the descent of the tree dismantles the heavy power lines that service one corner of Southern California. As the cables collapse the power fails in the city of La Habra.

The Monte Carlo enters a main intersection at the moment when the traffic signals fail. Simultaneously another car hurtles from the opposite direction. No moon, no other traffic. Street lights, signals, all visibility effaced by the weight of the tree that has fallen. The two cars meet, the Monte Carlo is hit broadside.

At 4:30 a.m. the telephone in the bedroom rings. Paul answers it.

"La Habra Community hospital," the phone sputters. "There's been an automobile accident and your daughter is being examined in the emergency ward. How soon can you get here?"

An extremely voluble Carol greets us, still shocked but entertaining her audience with descriptions of the moment of impact, the sounds of breaking glass and smashed metal, the frantic efforts to open the car door, the arrival of the paramedics. Sleepless, over-stimulated and eager to dramatize the event, all three young women sit in their assigned wheelchairs or race each other down the halls. A spontaneous undercurrent of laughter and satire.

Beneath Carol's left eye a purple bruise is forming. She shows us additional bruising on her left leg and right arm. She cannot forget the Monte Carlo and wants to see it again. "But I don't believe this; I just can't quit thinking about the car," she repeats, and so, before driving to the City of Hope, we stop by the garage where the crumpled automobile has been towed. "But it's totaled, totaled," Carol says incredulously, stepping past the wire fence and tugging at one of the door handles. "Daddy, that other car must have been really cooking!" Wide-eyed, she picks up some scattered hair pins and a splinter of glass from the dashboard. She is walking a bit stiffly. "Do you think anyone can put this automobile back together?"

"Honest, honey, I don't know about that, but I doubt it," Paul admits. The three of us share a deep reluctance to drive to the City of Hope. We dawdle alongside the door of the smashed car, exclaiming, commenting, postponing, as if time were at rest, the universe no longer in a state of action, and we three were suspended, mesmerized, in a small enclave of timelessness.

Dr. Kellon does not detain Carol for long, however. After an examination he merely says that the hematomas on her face and limbs are contained; and that she must return to the hospital for blood transfusions on Friday.

Easter Sunday. Carol comes to the house with Les. "Mother, I'm having chills," she says. "I just want to take a nice hot bath." She sluices hot water over herself and stands close to the electric wall heater in the bathroom.

"But, Carol," I protest, "I don't really believe this is the right thing to do for the hematoma." She is doctoring herself again, I think desperately. The thermometer reads 104 degrees. Chills and fever. I reach for the telephone.

Carol's friend Rick drives her to the City of Hope in the enormous camper that he has borrowed for the holiday trip to the Colorado river. A cluster of good friends goes along, sits beside her, stays near at hand during the admissions procedure, never a rapid process, and, this afternoon, endless.

They huddle together in the out-patient waiting room while a doctor is found who can examine her, someone else who can x-ray her. The hospital is understaffed. It is Easter, an inappropriate day for an emergency.

Carol clutches my hand, voiceless, looking angry, worried, resigned, annoyed. A nightmare is being played out before me in slow motion. No one can locate the hospital aides. The elevator jams on its way to the lab, stalls with Carol on a gurney and myself beside her. She is x-rayed incorrectly; the procedure has to be repeated. Walking in nightmare, attuning myself to the all-pervading lethargy, I tell my daughter's good friends, anxiously assembled around a coffee table, that she is to remain in the hospital. She will be treated for an infection. Some pain is as yet unaccounted for, but the x-rays have turned out satisfactory. Everyone is relieved and departs. Carol is wheeled to Wing Five, this time to a room near the nursing station. She grits her teeth. "So here I am, down where all the basket cases are being cared for," she says.

April 1. The day brings a heightened sense of mockery. Inexplicable changes occurring and rapidly, too, following the torpor of Easter Sunday. *A mediaeval mystery play*, I write in the diary, *a mocking mediaeval performance under the auspices of modern technology*. The scenes are not being acted out on the porch of some Thirteenth Century church, but are being run past like home movies, going by at an accelerated speed without explanation or proper commentary. The viewer is aware of confusion, contradictions, the flickers of irony. Sitting at Carol's bedside, I have to be both observer and commentator, finding the strands of meaning and piecing them together as best I can.

My daughter is being given pain pills, antibiotics, I.V.'s of cytosine and cytoxin, platelets, blood transfusions. Her left leg swells and inflames, red patches appear on her arms and chest, the bruise beneath the left eye darkens. Cold feet and hands. The nurses enlist me as another aide. I try both to warm Carol and to reduce the swelling. Ice packs, alcohol rubs, light massage.

Carol drifts into an entrancement as if a charm had been pronounced, a spell cast. She slips out of this bemusement only when visitors, her father, her sisters, come to talk and linger. Then she rallies, the brooding eyes kindle. When people leave, she glides under the enchantment again.

Someone makes a mistake. Carol is transported on a tall white gurney down cluttered halls and up to another floor for an abdominal examination. The order is cancelled. We reverse our path, proceed through the same halls past clinics and staring eyes. We meet Dr. Graham. Her eyes lock with mine and for an indefinable instant I see the taunting question in their depths: "You realize what this is at last, finally, don't you, Mrs. Trautmann?"

Dr. Kellon tells me cryptically that he suspects septicemia, blood poisoning. At one point he remarks that if and when the blood stabilizes he will continue the search for a bone marrow donor. Paul, agitated and angry, demands an interview with Kellon, wants to call in a specialist.

Carol delves deeper into her entrancement. "Mother, I want to go home. When can I go home?" She hesitates. "Yes, you know, you do know," she says, replying to my glance, the words I cannot utter. Fitfully phrases leave her mouth. I lean forward to hear them.

"The Monte Carlo. Well, you can make a motor bike out of it, maybe.... But how many cats do we have altogether now?"

The long pauses. The cup filled with its pineapple and lime drink remains steady in her clenched hand. "Where is Amy? What is Julie doing tonight?"

The warnings are being issued more and more frequently and from different doctors, Kellon and Fayhe and others. The blast cells are on the rise. You must expect the inevitable. But by now I am drawn completely within the circle of the entrancement and I do not hear the doctors. I barely see them move in and out of the small white room.

And still friends come to visit and talk and Carol rallies, sparkles for a moment before sinking back a little deeper under the spell. At last I cannot distinguish day from night, but during some ashen interval between the two, Carol whispers to me, "Mother, be my nurse." The kiss she gives me is dry, wrenched from chapped lips. "Mother, don't leave me."

I place a couple of chairs together, sleep next to her bed; for two nights I keep this post. During a dark midnight crisis I storm to the nurses' station. "My daughter is in pain, please give her a pain pill at once." The blank stares of the night nurses, head shaking, the puzzled consultation of charts. But can it be done without a doctor's sanction? Finally the request is met.

When morning arrives I begin my diary writing again. She notices and smiles. I start to sketch her profile upon white paper, attempting to reproduce the contour of the nose, the unruly hair, the smudged eyes, her hand as it grasps the cup, stays steady, stays poised.

The words I write in the diary break, fall apart, reach out for the inexpressible:

> ...to become my child, to pulse with her shallow
> breath
> feel with her, I am trying
> she needs me, she came from me once and is a part
> of me still
> turns to me now in her need and holds on
> even though she is saying nothing I hear her, 'you
> are there, mother...mother, where are you?'

I put down the diary and continue drawing, shadow and accent, knowing that I must create something during these hours—a poem, a sketch, a musical phrase—because creation is a part of the experience I witness: in my own fashion, out of my surest instinct, I must try to express what it is she now lives through. As the rhythms flow and ebb, I participate, I accompany my daughter:

> and I am with her   my love strong and deeply
> rooted
> perpetually growing
> my love asking 'how is it for you this moment, my

> child, where are you?'
> let nothing separate us
> am I not immersed in you   and you in me
> like the falling rain
> as it mingles with wind and leaves?

It is April 6, more rain and darkness. Paul stands at the window. We are all silent. Carol has not spoken for a long time. The room seems very white.

> be gentle with her, be kind, love her, enfold her
> may laughter surround her ears, may she hear it and
> be gladdened
> gladness sparkling through her shimmering form
> because
> she is a dance   a prism   an echoing chord of music
> beautiful in darkness
> foreign to pain
> new to transcendence

The white room is gray, the grayness of gauze drawn tight and pulled so as to form a screen. A vision is superimposed upon the gauze. I see the enactment of the ancient myth that is etched in memory, extending back through the ages, coursing down water and earth and moving like blood in the veins: the sacred valley, the cliff beside the sea toward which the grasses lean and the flowers decline, trembling upon their stems. The cliff split open by convulsion, avalanche and fire. The darkening sky, the silence. Into the hush rides the afterworld figure impelling the chariot and the pale imperious horses whose hooves smoke whenever they strike the ground. We cannot stop the horses from coming or prevent the iron arms of the charioteer from seizing the daughter, who, pinioned and constrained by a power she never summoned, turns away from us.

She descends, the chasm in the ground closes above her head, the valley's rift is sealed. Clouds of dust settle over the cliffs and the plain. The ocean is layered with dust and the mother's heart weighted with dust and bruised by the savage wind that blows across the earth heralding the time of grieving.

Carry it now, the burning branch of grief, not to be consumed by it, but to learn how life rises from the ashes. See again, with unmistakable joy, the innumerable and never-ending shapes of renascence.

Chapter 34

"It is no longer a policy of the City of Hope to plant trees as personal memorials," the official voice declaims emphatically. "Those eucalyptus trees around Hillquit were established many, many years ago."

After an interval of polite fencing my telephone call is transferred to the Los Angeles office of the administrative director whose brisk tones assure me, "Everything that *can* be done *will* be done." However, when I repeat my wish to plant a tree on the grounds, he objects with vigor. "It just isn't practical. It simply doesn't work out. We gave up the practice, oh, decades ago. We had to. The plaques hanging on the trunks get ruined; they become illegible. High winds tear out of the San Bernardino mountains sometimes and wreck the trees. People come back later, can't find their tree, and complain." He wants me to put up a plaque in Carol's name on a wall next to one of the wings, a pale green rectangle to blend with the hundreds of other rectangles.

I wait until he has run down. "I promised her a tree," I say. "It was a promise between us. I guess you could call it a commitment."

Silence. When he speaks again his tone has altered slightly. "I'm going to refer you to the superintendent of grounds, Mrs. Trautmann. You can discuss the matter further with him. What kind of a tree did you say you wanted to plant?"

"A lemon tree."

"A what?" Clearly the director does not find this choice suitable.

"A lemon tree," I insist. "Something with flowers and fruit. She...always liked lemons." An incomplete answer, I admit to myself, but there is a kind of reasoning behind it, a symbolism I do not wish to explain. A lemon tree because Carol loved tartness and spice and the color yellow. Carol, teasing us, pasting a strip of lemon rind across her teeth in a Halloween grin. The tang of lemon, sharp, stimulating, like Carol herself.

"...why don't you just donate money?" the director is saying.

Donations are another matter, I tell him firmly. They are not the issue here. "I promised her a tree," I repeat for the third time. "It's to be a living memorial, something vital." The choice of a lemon tree has already been decided upon, a group concensus in a way, the result of conversations with friends, Les and Debbie and others who remember Carol's distinct fondness for lemons. We have all agreed that no other tree will do.

The director says he must spend more time thinking and consulting on the matter. He calls me back an hour later. "Mr. Cameron, the grounds superintendent, will talk to you about the difficulties involved in planting a lemon tree," he says. "I suggest you get in touch with him right away."

To my complete surprise the superintendent, an experienced nurseryman from Canada, is amenable, capitulating almost at once to the idea of planting a tree as a memorial rather than buying a plaque.

"Quite a few people have given me money toward the purchase of this tree," I tell him, after we meet near the hospital parking lot. "It's an...oh, something they just want to do, to be included."

Mr. Cameron says yes, all right, that's good; but the main issue is the kind of tree, as well as the location, he adds thoughtfully. "But does it *have* to be a lemon tree?" he asks.

"No. I didn't promise her a lemon tree specifically. We just believe it's the sort of tree she would like." A shout is gathering inside me, a macabre impulse that I struggle to repress. Yes, lemons, a lemon tree! I want to scream. Some people in the world dote upon figs. Others chew betel nut or take snuff. Carol liked the bite of lemons.

"Ummmm...lemons?" he says as if reading my thought. "Yes, yes, I know. They're spicy—fragrant flowers and all that. But just let me tell you what happens to the fruit. It happens every single time in summer or fall, whenever the trees at this place begin to bear...Mostly we have avocados or peaches...Anyhow, people come in and just swarm over the lawns to pick off the fruit. And if they can't get the peach they're after, well, then they just tear off a branch."

He elaborates further, I listen and respond, but do not allow his arguments to deflect me. Our debate continues until at last the superintendent says, "Well, I really believe you are beginning to undermine me. I'll have to think it over a little bit longer, though, before I decide. Would you call me back on Monday?"

Monday morning, after the usual delays and re-routing at the switchboard, Mr. Cameron's voice finally reaches my ears. "I don't know exactly where we'll put that lemon tree yet, but your daughter's going to have one. But no plaque around the trunk," he cautions. "The plaques get torn off anyway. They're not worth it."

At the nursery in Whittier I am promised one Eureka lemon tree in a fifteen gallon can, about seven feet high, already bearing lemons and yellow winter leaves that will turn darker green in time. Delivery will take two weeks, enough time certainly for the selection of an appropriate site.

Joyce accompanies me once again to the City of Hope and meets the superintendent. The three of us stroll about the grounds examining possible locations. Quite a number of new buildings are being constructed near the main entrance—among these a separate division for young people which is to be called the Familian Children's Center. We unanimously choose this part of the research complex for a site. "Right here against the north wall," Mr. Cameron announces, indicating a rather muddy area littered with bits of broken cement. "This will be just fine."

The actual tree planting ceremony takes place on a warm day in June. A circle of people gathers, poetry is read, Dr. Ed Bloomfield speaks to us about hope, the word, the hospital, and "the hope that before this tree reaches its full stature a cure will be found for the illness that took Carol from us." Paul and I are the first to shovel dirt around the tree's roots. Others pick up the spade and throw on more soil. The tree is planted.

The last time I visited Carol's tree I observed that it now stands on the circumference of a children's playground and is part of a border of greenery that shelters behind a strong metal fence.

Leukemic children and infants suffering from catastrophic illness are no longer sequestered on a roof top. They play in a large circle of sand edged by a concrete sidewalk; and they can choose from among a fine selection of playground equipment that includes a jungle gym made of logs, a sheet metal slide and a large rubber tire swing. The circle of sand and the collar of cement both sweep past the lemon tree. A few toy plastic cars and digging spoons are scattered near its slender trunk.

The branches shiver softly, laden with their yellow and dark green leaves; several small green globes, the rind just beginning to turn golden, swing freely in the depths of Carol's tree. It is still the only lemon tree on the grounds, more than doubled in height, and daily growing taller.

SYCAMORE CANYON

The hillside at my back door is part of a larger slope that rises to a crest, levels, then rises again to form the second hump of the Bactrian camel-backed hill overlooking Sycamore Canyon. The canyon itself, although blocked and rendered invisible by the undulations of the earth and by dark avocado orchards, exists as a vital element in our lives, being not only the distant background against which we move, but also the nucleus from which the hills periodically allow their occupants to make brief raids upon the surrounding civilization that threatens from every angle. Over the years we experience intermittent visits from a variety of dwellers in the earth.

During a dry September snakes sometimes cross over driveways and roads in their search for water. Usually the rattlesnakes invade the homes higher up on the hill, while the less intimidating gopher and garter snakes penetrate back yards and patios farther down. Skunks also saunter around the houses at these lower levels, once in a while colonizing in abandoned garages. Opossums, racoons, the cottontail rabbit, even the coyote, make occasional forays. While deer seldom encroach upon human territory, they can often be seen grazing just across the canyon where they blend nicely with the red-brown soil and the chaparral.

The heart of the hills still vibrates with a life of its own, for these ridges make up a spur of the San Gabriel mountains which, in turn, are linked to the towering Sierra Nevada. We are not true mountain climbers and remain in awe of the aloof snow-covered peaks which we seldom visit, but the hills envelop us, we live within and upon them, are keenly aware of their seasonal patterns and shifts in color and configuration. We are drawn to the hills because of their variety, the strength and depth of their unfathomable silences.

Many canyons furrow the hills but Sycamore Canyon is the one we know best. Because it has been designated a bird sanctuary, the valley reverberates with the twittering calls of hundreds of birds that settle down among the shrubs or fly from one leafy support to another, streaking the air crimson, blue, silver and pale yellow like crayon marks rapidly erased. A continual colloquy goes on among the birds, an unending dialogue that is silenced only when human beings stagger down the second hump of the camel-shaped hill to land on the canyon floor, crashing or sliding along one of the scanty trails and clinging to tall weeds for support.

Amy, Carol, Julie and I made this difficult descent a number of times during our first decade in California. We never considered ourselves genuine bird-watchers, but were conscious always of the uneasy darting life that quivered and vocalized around us, that remained hushed for long intervals after our loud arrival in the valley. The birds, we used to remark, like to stay in hiding; they are secretly watching *us*, the explorers, for we thought of ourselves as members of an expedition in a wilderness terrain.

Like all serious adventurers we carried concentrated rations—chocolate, dried fruit, small apples and bottles of water. We picked up large branches from the ground and used them as staves to aid us in climbing up or down the canyon walls. Each of us developed a technique for hugging the topsoil of steep slides and for digging in with her heels. When the sun was at the zenith we dropped below the dusty road slanting to the east and followed the parallel course of the thin brook which purred within narrow banks lined by the bent rusty sycamores that give the canyon its name.

"We're survivors, aren't we?" Carol remarked one warm morning as we trudged beside the tree-shaded stream, trying to keep up with its constant changes of pace and shape.

"We sure are," her sisters replied in unison. One of them added: "Yes, but could we please find a spot along here to rest for a little while? It's hot enough."

Amy went out ahead, racing back soon to describe the territory we were about to enter. We stumbled onto a small beach of mud and stones where the banks rose sharply and the earth was eroding from around the sycamores, leaving countless exposed tree roots that were intertwined and twisted like serpents. "How weird," Carol and Julie chimed together as they stared at the coils and tangles.

"Well, do we really want to stay *here*?" I asked.

"Sure," Amy said, climbing on one of the larger roots. "Why not? Feel how cool the air is—and feel all this soft clay. It's great."

And so we discovered Root Camp, moved in, ate our raisins and apples, lay down to rest, first cooling our perspiring feet in the running water which was transparently clear at the center and brackish with leaves and decaying seed pods at the edges. The twisted tree roots were reduced at once from the grotesque to the merely strange and functional; we hung our damp socks on them. We stretched out on the clay beach and drowsed, listening to frogs and insects, the far away clapping of a cow bell. "Hey, let's make this our permanent base of operations," I heard someone mutter before falling asleep.

After the winter rains pelted the hillsides for weeks on end we would find Root Camp nearly immersed in torrents. March and April were the wild months. The serpentine columns of roots strained whatever flooded past them, caught and kept battered dragon flies, tail feathers, blossoms, drowned rodents, plastic cups and paper bags, the flotsam left by the storms. In early autumn when the sun attained an almost paralyzing force, the stream went dry, or was diminished to a trickle, flanked by naked sycamore roots that shone silvery and gargantuan like carvings or archaic statues within the valley of the Nile. Regardless of the season Root Camp established itself as our base. We ate here, planned and disagreed and discussed the relative size and position of the canyon's principal topographical features.

Each of us could enumerate the valley's most noteworthy landmarks: the windings of the dusty road that skirted the stream; the hollow tree which everyone climbed, using boards some earlier pioneer nailed years ago across the trunk as ladder rungs; the bee log with its colony of honey bees set in a meadow of wild flowers; the cave high up on a sheer wall tantalizingly out of reach; fenced-in areas where cows from a neighboring dairy were still brought to pasture; the swamp far east of Root Camp at the point where the dusty road contracted and changed to the barest of trails. The road, in fact, terminated at this swamp which became the culmination of all our investigative efforts. The thick stagnant waters in the marsh resonated with the harsh commentaries of frogs; its edges bristled with rushes and the brown velvet spikes of cattails. Having arrived at this destination, Carol would invariably try to capture a frog at the swamp's border, but the raucous creatures were too quick for her.

"I want a frog to take home," she told me once. "I'll put it in the triangle at the side of the house and keep the hose running so it won't miss the swamp so much." And then, "Mom, what do you suppose they're saying?" she asked wonderingly as the frogs increased the volume and dissonance of their outraged croaking.

Beyond the swamp on the other side of the next slope that peaks gently to the north lies a section of land belonging to the far-ranging cemetery known as Rose Hills. One hot summer afternoon we circled the swamp and stepped over the boundary line into the cemetery grounds. We threw ourselves down among the weeds and gazed at the pattern of roads lying beneath us, the maze of markers reflecting the sunlight. A dozen large bulldozers were parked close by. Although abandoned and driverless, the big yellow machines suggested a waiting army and seemed a potential threat to the canyon we had just traversed.

Julie made an angry gesture. "They better stay parked right here," she said, pointing.

"Yeah," Carol agreed abruptly.

"They better leave our camp and Sycamore Canyon alone." Amy shook her finger at the twelve motionless machines.

Without more words we turned our backs on the bulldozers and hiked down the trail onto the road, greeting the familiar landmarks by name as we passed them and taking satisfaction in their permanency, progressing from swamp to cave to hollow tree until we arrived at the foot of the tall slope that we must scale in order to regain civilization. Before we began the ascent, hauling ourselves up by means of sticks and whatever large obliging plants we could grasp, Carol scribbled a note on a piece of paper which she then stuffed into a tiny blue bottle, one of the many treasures she liked to carry loose in her pockets. She capped the bottle and hurled it at the stream just beneath our feet.

"What in the world are you doing?" I asked her.

"That's a message. It's secret," she said mysteriously. "It's a letter to the frogs and next year when the rains are over I'm going to hike out and find the bottle again in the swamp."

"You think the frogs will answer?" I asked. "Carol, wherever do you get these ideas? How can you be sure that blue bottle is going to make it all the way to the swamp?"

"It will, you'll see," she answered, starting to scramble up through the weeds and chaparral.

But she doesn't go back next year. None of us returns. The months pass, the hills change color many times, green to bronze to purple-gray; they are seared by the sun, drenched with rain, burnished a rich gold in spring because of the wild mustard that blooms and spreads out a shining mantle, then pales and withers to straw.

Months stretch into years. The three remaining survivors of our team of explorers never visit the canyon. I doubt if any of us will descend to the valley floor again, climb the hollow tree or cool her feet in the stream beneath the sycamores. Yet, as the years pass, I walk frequently across the two humps of the familiar hill, noticing the processes of change, what revives every season, what declines and vanishes. Carol's dog Blackie accompanies me. Together we stand on the second crest high above the canyon floor gazing down at the sycamores and the dusty road.

The hills below always captivate me. My eyes follow their sweeping advance to the north and the east. On certain days I consider their softness, how they fold and melt into one another, the sense of fusion this involvement conveys; at other times, especially in the evenings under a bright moon, I find them exacting, separatist, every detail of thistle and cactus and foot-path emergent as if etched on a silver plate.

I know where I am when I stand at the top of the hill,

just as I know the location of each remembered landmark within the depths of the canyon. If I continue going west along the asphalt road under my feet, I shall come to a point where I can look across the valley and see a group of black trees through which the illuminated sign ROSE HILLS is glowing and evoking the illusion of a dark irregularly shaped mansion lighted from within by rosy fires. If I stoop beneath a section of barbed wire and walk to the east, I can watch the straggling trees along the canyon bottom gradually dwindle and blend into the far-off reaches of the swamp. But I do not really know if the swamp still exists or if the yellow bulldozers have destroyed it. I can only speculate whether the sluggish waters, grown even darker with algae and black-green bullrushes, are keeping the tiny blue bottle that contains Carol's message to the frogs.

Often I stand upon the summit moving neither to the west or to the east. Instead I linger in between these two compass points, visualizing Root Camp's position almost directly opposite me, secluded, of course, by trees and underbrush, but invisibly present just below the distant powdery road. Root Camp hangs upon a fulcrum, is a balance, a place where I pause and refresh myself. Across the hushed canyon it sends out an almost tangible comfort, becoming more and more of a sanctuary to me now, a restless woman exploring many worlds.

THE COMPANION

One of my favorite walks takes me to an acre or so of untamed ground, a stretch of level plain that juts out high above the city where I live. The earth tangles and bunches here in great knots of wildflowers and aloes. A few small trees struggle up from the hard adobe. This is the site I imagine Carol choosing for her own house, a cottage with rough ivory-colored bricks and a red tiled roof. The mortar which cements the building has been applied so casually that it oozes from the edges of the bricks like thick vanilla cream. A jacaranda tree rains purple flowers across the roof tiles, a tropical rice-paper plant sways at the front door. White and purple daisies over the lawn. Firethorn bushes and ferns.

I stand below the window of Carol's house, musing, and the companion stands alongside me. She is exceedingly old this morning, old in the sense of centuries, not years, and she wears both the garments and the demeanor of an ancient wise-woman, one who might be, perhaps, an interpreter of the oracles in the forests of Epirus or a guardian of sacred shrines during those years before the arrival of the sun god from Asia. Her robes and cowl are blue. The face that is tilted toward my own crinkles expressively into a network of countless tiny lines. The lustrous eyes are deepset under a prominent forehead. Ancient and wrinkled though she may be, her steps spring lightly.

The staff in her hand inscribes a sweeping arc that ends at the cottage window. We both look into the room overhead and see my daughter on the opposite side of the glass. Carol is sitting upon an oval braided rug playing jack-straws with her two small children. I am close enough to see their dark hazel eyes and to follow the ambling awkward gait of the furry kitten that rolls from one child to the other. Carol picks up the kitten and drops it on her own knee; when the small animal begins to climb, clinging tenaciously to the corduroy cloth, she laughs. The sound echoes faintly, like crystals cupped and held jingling within two muted hands.

The companion smiles at me, a long slow smile that

engages every wrinkle and plane of her parchment face. Carol throws a ball up toward the ceiling of the room which hovers a moment and disappears. Instantly she goes after it, slipping out the front door past the rice-paper plant and running on swift noiseless feet.

"Where is she going?" I ask, but the walkway underneath me swings forward simultaneously, its composition changing without effort into a concrete sidewalk. We are borne past traffic and tall buildings until we reach the center of a large city. It is the rush hour and I have lost sight of Carol; but all at once she reappears on the corner opposite us waiting for the traffic signal to turn green. She wears a long black gown that flaps around her ankles. One hand holds tight to a rolled-up paper which she alternately brandishes and examines closely. When the light changes she strides toward me.

"She's searching for you, too," the companion says quietly. And now I hear my daughter calling: "Mother, mother, I've got something to show you. Just look at this—" The paper flourishes above her head, her widened eyes probe through the hastening crowds.

"She has passed the bar examination at last," my interpreter informs me, "and she wants to tell you just what it was like."

I begin to shout and wave my arms. She rushes across the street, draws closer, approaches, and then veers off course. The streets dip and narrow, the buildings change to high-rising slopes and the sidewalk becomes a dirt trail. Soon we are deep within the mountains. Carol is just ahead of us, hiking rapidly, easing the strap of her knapsack as she goes. She comes full stop at the bottom of a gully, glances around as if analyzing the terrain, bends down, sinking slightly into the bed of a dried-up stream. She fingers the gravel deposited by the once-flowing waters and carefully examines the pebbles, sorting them out, keeping only two objects: a rock containing the imprint of a fossil fern and a piece of rose quartz which she holds high to reflect the sunlight. I observe how both her sunburned wrists are free of the shadowy stipple of the I.V. She sets her two finds inside the compartments of a small plastic carrying case.

I consider her movements, the intent look on her face. "Oh, that's what it is, then. I see." My words reverberate thinly across still air. "What she really, secretly wants to become is a geologist, isn't that the truth?"

No one answers. I look uncertainly at my guide who is leaning on her staff. Two blue jays lift from the live oaks and spiral upward. I watch their flight, lower my gaze and discover that Carol has gone. The companion motions, leads me past dun hills covered with underbrush onto an expanse of beach. Spray meets us, hissing as it breaks free and dances over the curled edges of the waves. The cliffs nearby are honey-combed with sea caves, some of them under water, others resting on sand right above the seething ocean. The cave my guide decides to enter occupies a precarious portion of the tideline. A low surge of foam pursues us and spills an arabesque across the cavern floor when it recedes.

Opposite us, at a considerable distance and close to a towering wall, Carol sits in a shaft of blue twilight, her head bent above the sewing materials on her lap. There is an overflow of coarse squares of canvas at her feet, folders of embroidery needles and bundles of colored thread. Carol sews. The threads, as she pulls and loosens them from their coils, throb with animation, living fibers of scarlet and turquoise, purple and amber. A slim needle flashes in her hand, sweeps through the square of material she is holding and traces a whirlwind of color upon the pallid cloth. She sews with the rapidity of moving light. The mound of squares beside her, embroidered and evidently completed, heightens.

"What is she sewing?" I ask. My question provokes no echo at all within the huge cave.

"Pictures," is the reply I receive.

"Yes, but of what?"

"Oh, the future." The companion pauses. "And the past and the present, too. It is all the same."

"Whose future? What past? How can they be the same?"

Carol hears me. She looks into the mouth of the cave and sees me. At once she waves delightedly and holds up the tapestried square she is working on. I am able to perceive only a glimmer of coppery gold and an impression of bright sweeping lines. She blows me a kiss.

The gestures she makes across the dividing distance appear to mime her thought; but even without them I would understand. The focus of her mind engages my own: *See, I've known all along that you were here. The barriers are really very weak, flimsier than you imagine. And what do they matter? A thing like invisibility, only a trick, a jest...the thoughts leap and tumble toward me.*

She lifts up another brilliant square of cloth. I step closer. But the tide is in, pounding at our backs. The ripple that teased the cave's floor as we entered now swells into a large wave and fills the cavern with thundering sound. A wall of water builds quickly, passes the companion and me, rises, paints over Carol's form with rapid blue-green strokes. Through their translucence I can still perceive my daughter's steady gaze, the warmth of her attention, the moving gleaming needle in her hand.

Gradually I am led outside the sea cave. Fragrant humid air like that permeating a greenhouse and the tang of brine surround us. The path we now walk upon seems to lie through water meadows, but it has grown so dark I am not certain. Everywhere the blackness of the unseen and unlighted sea bed, the continual rhythmical flowing on either side of the course we follow.

The companion sheds a radiance upon the sea surge. Her silver hair is like a phosphorescent net of filaments that lengthen and filter through the shoals. Her hands reach deep into the black and blueblack depths. As if she were plucking flowers she brings together an assortment out of the dark void, choosing from among its delicate structures a minute spray of stars, a sprig of planets just born, a miniature budding sun, a rare white-gold blossoming moon.

"For you," she breathes. Gently she assembles this bouquet from the illimitable gardens.

I instruct my fear to be invisible
mute and deaf
but fear
skips alongside me the instant I wake and stammers:
"…if I lose you…if I lose you…if I lose you"
and cocks its elongate ears
toward each splintering second of uncertainty
and listens, listens
becomes the world's acrobat   performing before crowds
walks a tightrope   through the slow afternoons
changing at six o'clock sharp
into the long distance runner
who will leave messages
hourly
during the night
at the door
of my brain

my wasted hours
are like water
running from a faucet
over my fingers
droplets
that I want to collect
in a silver cup
and give
you
to drink

we do little but bring you flowers   one more armful
another procession of colors to fill up gray space
we hand you floral gestures
peppermint-striped carnations
our bland pink roses, our cheerful autumn asters
never thinking
how you must hate the flowers   how tired you grow
longing for health and life   not more flowers

ah, the flowers
are seeding my vision
I dream you   fresh gold   exquisite
blossoming with the sun's eloquence
and the clear proud logic of darkness

there is no more time left for subterfuge
the turning wheel   has put on
iron spikes
and is rotating
across me

I am being diminished
under this tread

unless the subject for discussion
is pain
let no one speak
to me
now

afterwards
thinking to take a bit of you with them
friends divide up the pottery you fashioned in ceramics class
having thrown the clay blithely
laughing at your own raw awkwardness
in learning this new skill

one friend takes the pinch pot
somebody else acquires a vase   then a jar goes
the bowls disappear
I don't mind
months ago you gave me a heavy cup that shows your finger
    marks
on the inside of its smoky rim
and one small flower vase which attempts a blue glaze
'well, it's supposed to be blue, mom," you said 'do you
really like it, do you really?'
you repeat   standing irresolutely at the door of my room
pleading and unsure
ready to walk away from me forever
leaving me these polished pieces of yourself

never have the hills been more green
never has the sun haloed them more clearly
never have the blue shadows looked more inviting
never have the doves spoken more confidingly
never have the clouds moved with more distinction
never has the wind blown with more passion
never have I longed more for the sight of you
than on this day in April

your grave is a rumpled brown handkerchief

at the borders where the shaggy grass is catching on
people scatter their pocket contents   a marigold
a rosebud   a match   a cigarette   a damp pink ribbon

within the prim company you keep these days
headstones and urns and hedges
your space alone seems disheveled
littered by these several odd mementoes
jangled together discordantly
as if spilled out by the same rude gesture
that brought you to this place and
dropped you here   protesting

Carol, I keep your dancing shoes
at the bottom of the closet still
the ones you bought and were never able to use
for the class in acrobatic dancing
you were never able to begin
I dust the shoes sometimes
and turn them around the points of the compass
setting them down at north north east
or wherever I think
you might be dancing now

I am locked into these hills
as surely as the clay being metamorphosed
into adobe   into granite
given a million years or so
given me, my bones
mortared and mixed with the bones of rabbits
and coyotes
the frail leavings of spiders and cactus spines
locked into these potpourri hills
my stoniness, your grace

'mother, I want to live life as a duck some day'
you told me once
it was a joke   of course
but hide-and-seek has become a game I take seriously
and, shape-changer, among your many metamorphoses
is this rainbow-mallard swimming toward the banks
carrying the sun on its slender neck
escorted by wood ducks at either side

your beak sieves water
your feet trail sapphire
you dive and disappear in one swift continuous movement

I am breathless
the anticipation of returning
paralyzes me   I am unable to step from this fixed shoreline

O   when you break through the waves again, shape-changer
what will you look like
who will you be?

Books From Cleis Press

THE ABSENCE OF THE DEAD
IS THEIR WAY OF APPEARING
Mary Winfrey Trautmann
ISBN: 0-939416-04-2
8.95

WOMAN-CENTERED PREGNANCY
AND BIRTH
Ginny Cassidy-Brinn, R.N., Francie Hornstein,
Carol Downer & the Federation of Feminist
Women's Health Centers
ISBN: 0-939416-03-4
11.95

VOICES IN THE NIGHT:
WOMEN SPEAKING ABOUT INCEST
ed. Toni A.H. McNaron & Yarrow Morgan
ISBN: 0-939416-02-6
7.95

FIGHT BACK! FEMINIST RESISTANCE
TO MALE VIOLENCE
ed. Frédérique Delacoste & Felice Newman
ISBN: 9-939416-01-8
13.95

ON WOMEN ARTISTS: POEMS 1975–1980
Alexandra Grilikhes
ISBN: 0-939416-00-X
4.95